# Master Your Stress

You can't always avoid stressful environments, but you can take an active role in making sure stress doesn't control your life. Let *Mastery of Stress* be your first step toward a healthier and happier lifestyle. With the help of an authentic Master of Yoga, you'll quickly embrace the yoga-inspired techniques in this book to:

- Restore flagging concentration and interrupt the flow of repetitive, obsessive, or unwelcome thoughts

- Increase the amount and quality of energy and vitality available to you at work and at home

- Access your deep reserves of creativity while providing periods of cellular and psychological rest and restoration

- Flush out toxins and metabolic by-products that drain your energy and lower your resistance to disease

- Produce a sense of calm, centering, and well-being

- Adjust and balance the flow of energy in the acupuncture meridians

- Alter brain chemistry, balance your nervous system, and alleviate states of anger and anxiety

- Significantly increase fine motor control

Take a few minutes out of your day and learn to master your stress—it's easy with this helpful guide.

## About the Author

Paul Skye (Australia) works as a stress management consultant and yoga teacher. Formerly initiated as Swami Ajnananda Saraswati in India in 1977, he was the director of the Tasmanian Yoga Therapy Centre from 1988 to 1993, and was formally recognized as a Master of Yoga by Paramahamsa Niranjananda of the world's first government-approved Yoga University in Bihar, India.

## To Write to the Author

If you wish to contact the author or would like more information about this book, please write to the author in care of Llewellyn Worldwide and we will forward your request. Both the author and publisher appreciate hearing from you and learning of your enjoyment of this book and how it has helped you. Llewellyn Worldwide cannot guarantee that every letter written to the author can be answered, but all will be forwarded. Please write to:

Paul Skye
c/o Llewellyn Worldwide
P.O. Box 64383, Dept. K630-0
St. Paul, MN 55164-0383, U.S.A.

Please enclose a self-addressed stamped envelope for reply, or $1.00 to cover costs. If outside U.S.A., enclose international postal reply coupon.

*PAUL ❖ SKYE*

# MASTERY
# OF
# STRESS

*Techniques for Relaxation
in the Workplace*

1998
Llewellyn Publications
St. Paul, Minnesota 55164-0383
U.S.A.

FIRST EDITION
First Printing, 1998

Cover design: Lisa Novak
Interior illustrations: Carrie Westfall
Thanks to Wende Lee Weiss, and the author
   for providing original sketches, which the illustrations were based on.
Book design and editing: Michael Maupin

**Library of Congress Cataloging-in-Publication Data**
Skye, Paul, 1944 –
   Mastery of stress : techniques for relaxation in the workplace / Paul Skye.
      p.  cm.
   Includes index.
   ISBN 1-56718-630-0
   1. Stress management. 2. Job stress. 3. Yoga, Hatha.
RA785.S55 1998
613.7'046—dc21                                              98-34005
                                                               CIP

Llewellyn Publications
A Division of Llewellyn Worldwide, Ltd.
P.O. Box 64383, Dept. K630-0
St. Paul, MN 55164-0383, U.S.A.

Printed in the United States of America.

## DEDICATION

TO SOME 53 YEARS of "hard travel-ing" and Woody Guthrie. A friend once told me that Woody, when told that someone had stolen one of his songs, replied: "He's a fool; he only steals from me. I've stolen from everybody."

To all the friends, helpers and colleagues from whom I've stolen freely and joyfully, but most of all:

To Gurudev Paramahamsa Satyananda, formerly of Bihar School of Yoga, India; from whom I could not steal, because he has given everything I could take. Paramahamsa Satyananda Saraswati is con-sidered to be one of the greatest living authorities on the Science of Yoga. He is currently retired and living in relative seclusion in Bihar.

# CONTENTS

# FIGURES & PRACTICES

# The Essential Mastery of Stress

IN 1966, I VISITED the Tibetan Refugee Center in Darjeeling, Northern India, with Angela, the woman who was to become my wife and companion for over ten years. We stayed in a hotel with the retired chief magistrate of the tiny Himalayan kingdom of Assam. We quickly became good friends and spent many hours each evening discussing everything from the current international situation, to the cultural richness of the Indian subcontinent.

He introduced us to the science of yoga and took great care to distinguish the practical and therapeutic value of the centuries-old techniques from the mythological cultural fabric into which it had become woven. He saw yoga as a pure science of human potential and insisted that it be brought to Western society as a suitable panacea for the problems facing it.

Over the next ten years, Angela and I lived in Tasmania, Australia, and explored yoga and meditation until, in December 1976, she suffered a fatal brain hemorrhage, the result of a small congenital malformation of one of the blood vessels in her brain. From the moment she had the stroke until she died six days later, I remained with her as much as possible. While she was being transferred from the hospital in Northern Tasmania to the intensive care unit of the hospital in Hobart, something happened that changed my life.

A friend drove me in his car, following the ambulance to the hospital. I had been without sleep for four days, and I felt exhausted and powerless. My friend played some Gregorian chants on the car tape deck and told me to recline my seat and get some rest. As I lay back and closed my eyes, I remembered a phrase from my yoga studies. "When the student is ready, then the master will appear." So I mentally prayed "If there's a master out there, if I'm not ready now—I never will be. Please tell me what to do, because I've got no resources left. I'm empty."

Instantly I heard a very clear voice, perfectly enunciated, say, "Contact Swami Satyavedananda in Hobart!" I thought to myself, *Okay, I'll do it.* As soon as we reached the city, I made some inquiries and found that this man taught yoga at a small center in a beach-side suburb. He was asked to come to the hospital and duly arrived.

I immediately noticed he was a tall man with a shaven head, and he was swathed in deep burnt-orange robes. He projected an air of quiet reserve. From the time of the Swami's visit, everything changed. Over the five days following her stroke, Angela regained and lost consciousness intermittently and, each time she awoke, she was confused and terrified. She had no recollection of what had happened and awoke in strange surroundings, partially paralyzed and unable to talk. We had worked out a code of eye blinks for communication and, during these last hours of her life, I felt all her love and concern. Each time she regained consciousness, I was there to explain the situation and to comfort her. She was particularly upset about our young son Hal, who she was still breastfeeding. She was perfectly at peace in herself and her eyes told a story far more intense than our crude system could convey. The Swami, who had trained in India, was able to help Angela come to a point of peace, total clarity, and acceptance which remained with her right up to the moment she died.

As he left the hospital, the Swami had said, "Come and see me when things are better," so some weeks later I went to visit him at his center. He suggested that I join one of his yoga classes, but I politely declined, explaining that I was quite happy with my own practice of ten years. I said to him, "Look, I'm really grateful for the help you gave, but I really don't want to get involved with any sect or cult, and I definitely don't want to have anything to do with orange robes and shaven heads!"

At this, he threw his head back, roaring with laughter, and said, "Good, good—keep a healthy skepticism!" He then suggested that I might like to join one of his meditation classes. I thought for a few moments. I had been practicing transcendental meditation (TM) for eight years, and although I felt I received a lot of benefit from the technique, I suspected that there was much more to be experienced and explored, so I agreed.

After regularly attending the class for about six months, he said to me, "My guru is coming to Australia in a few weeks and I thought that maybe you would like to meet him." I told him I'd think about it. My reason dictated that if this man whose accomplishments and knowledge I had come to respect and admire had been trained by his guru, it would make good sense to "go to the top."

On July 4, 1977, I met Swami Satyananda, the guru of my teacher. The moment he spoke, I recognized the voice I had heard in the car on the way to the hospital in Hobart six months before. I can't describe the emotions I felt at that point. He initiated me into a meditation technique, and then said, "You should come and be a Swami with me in India."

By late October of that year, I sold my full-time Naturopathic practice, gave away all of my property (including a farm of 120 acres) and was on my way to India. I was initiated as a Swami (which simply means "master of one's self") on December 1, 1977, and suddenly found myself with my head shaved and my only possessions my orange robes.

I remained in the ashram until May the following year, when Swami Satyananda sent me to give a lecture tour of Southeast

Asia. During that time I worked in the International Yoga Research Coordinating Center with several Australian medical doctors who were also Swamis.

The whole thrust of our research was to understand and explain the application of classical yoga techniques on the management of the vast range of disease that afflicts modern society. This was "yoga therapy," and much of what I assimilated there, by living and breathing an atmosphere of dedicated research and yoga practice, stripped of its veil of confusing allegory and superstition, forms the basis of this Mastery of Stress program.

Over the past eighteen years as a stress management consultant and yoga teacher, I have had many doctors, psychiatrists, and psychologists as clients, students, and friends. The role of stress to illness has become increasingly well defined for all of us, as has the value of the yoga techniques in relieving that stress. The journey has been an exciting and fulfilling one as I have gone on to practice and instruct in a field I'm certain will help to lay the foundation for a society truly well equipped to meet the demands of the future.

My observations and experience have resulted in an answer to the single crucial question to which I've given the name the Essential Mastery of Stress. It is essential both because it is greatly needed and because it approaches the question intimately, educationally, and practically. I've chosen the word "mastery" rather than "management" because I'm certain that we can incorporate all that stress has to teach us and use our innate potential to rise to the challenge of mastering its effects.

I hope you use the methods, and enjoy the journey, too.

Paul Skye
Brisbane, Australia
November 1998

# CHAPTER 1

# The Business of Stress
# (or, It's a Stressful Business)

THERE'S A STORY OF a man who had to cross a stream in a small boat with his three possessions: a lion, a goat, and a bale of hay. The boat was very small and could only accommodate the man and one possession at a time. What could he do? If he took the hay, the lion would eat the goat. If he took the lion, the goat would eat the hay.

After some deliberation, he bundled the goat into the boat and crossed the stream, leaving her on the other side. He then returned and picked up the hay. When he reached the goat, he dumped the hay on the shore, picked up the goat and returned to the starting point. He dropped off the goat, then made the crossing with the lion, leaving it safely with the bale of hay. He returned for the goat, finally arriving with all three intact on the far shore.

*The man dealt with this stressful challenge successfully, even providing himself with some physical exertion, with all the rowing and lifting.*

Success in dealing with this situation came from the intelligent and rational manipulation of the *external* elements, the environmental factors. On the other hand....

Once upon another time (could be yesterday, today, or tomorrow), Margaret was an executive with a very difficult job to do. She had to rise early, as her home was a long way from the big city, and

1

finish all her domestic duties by 7.00 A.M., and then drive for an hour and a half in hectic, life-threatening traffic to reach her office early enough to make several important phone calls to a different time zone.

Six months earlier, she had been passed over for the job of general manager of her division, a promotion she had expected and wanted for the last four years. Margaret now had to answer to the very upwardly mobile man, *twelve years her junior*, who had beaten her out of the promotion. During this time, the new general manager had significantly changed the work environment, redefining areas of responsibility and accountability and instituting new practices.

Margaret now shared her position with another executive, after her new boss had explained that, while he appreciated that she had been doing her best to cope with an ever-increasing workload, he felt that the position was better fulfilled by the appointment of an additional colleague who would also "help to give a wider perspective."

Since these changes, she had experienced what seemed to be a never-ending succession of minor respiratory tract infections and her digestion, which had never been good, had deteriorated to the point where she was in constant discomfort. Her physician prescribed diagnostic procedures that revealed she had colon cancer. She underwent surgery and made a full and complete recovery. She eventually left the job, and she and her husband sold their house and purchased a small farm. At last report, she and her family were doing fine.

I have chosen the happy ending, but the reality is that most of these scenarios, which are all too common, don't end that way at all. This was a stressful situation Margaret couldn't address by the intelligent and rational manipulation of the *external* elements. She had no control over the events in the workplace. Ultimately she changed her situation, but many people either don't recognize that possibility or, even if they do, feel unable to act so drastically. Many die "in the harness." Much can be done. Much *must* be done. Stress, improperly addressed, is a killer: a killer of bodies, minds, aspirations, and companies.

When it comes to *effective* stress management, there are a great many programs that promise much and fail miserably to deliver in the long term. Most of them depend heavily on attitudinal manipulations, "reconditioning," a high level of personal dynamism in the presentation, and usually, game playing of various types. These programs can be "dangerous," and they are usually very expensive. After implementation, senior management feels that they have made a significant investment and that all ought to be well from that point on. The attitude persists that, if the company provided the program, and the results are not forthcoming, it must somehow be the fault of the participants. The problems have not been solved, but the company feels it has done what was required to address the question.

But there are no quick fixes. The reality is that we, as a society, are overwhelmed by occupational, environmental, mental, emotional, domestic, and dietary stress. Psychology seems the most effective tool we have, because we perceive stress in the province of the mind. Although mind, attitudes, and preferences are certainly involved, stress can be more accurately described in the dimension of the *body*—in the brain itself, in the organs, in the musculature. It is the physical body that reflects the effects of stress, in impaired functioning of the vehicle for the mind.

An integrated, ongoing stress management program addressing all aspects of the human being—body, mind, and spirit—and the way in which the physical workplace affects these dimensions—can enhance performance and increase productivity. In terms of corporate and individual longevity and efficiency, such a program can make the difference between the "player" and the "stayer." Ongoing is critical because it is essential for stress management to be so integrated into the fabric of all business and personal endeavor that it becomes part of the basic structure, the everyday routine, of business and life.

## MANAGEMENT: SURVIVAL AND SUCCESS

A company's recognition of the necessity for effective stress management, from boardroom to frontline, will be one of the most significant determinants of that company's survival and, more importantly, success.

Until now, management has really been playing catch-up where this question is concerned. Few general managers and even fewer boards of directors have had a good hard look at the impact that stress is having and, more importantly, will have on the corporate future.

There is already a huge building tide of cumulative corporate stress that goes unaddressed in the form of cutbacks, downsizing, and lay-offs. Talented and productive people are swamped by this inexorable wave, and, as they go under, the load on those remaining or newly recruited to replace them increases. The scenario of mature and responsible adults hiding in their offices, crying in washrooms, drowning their senses in alcohol, or simply not turning up for work because they can't face another day is a real one and it is already here.

The impact of stress on the health and vitality of the individual is directly and financially reflected in the health and vitality of the company. The full impact of the underlying hidden cost, both personal and corporate, of an inefficient or short-sighted approach to stress management will become increasingly apparent over the next decade. From the company's point of view, by the time someone goes on stress leave or goes under with a stress-related disease (and here we include conditions such as repetitive colds and flu, heart disease, migraine headaches, high blood pressure, asthma, insomnia, ulcers, and cancer), the condition has already produced significant cost in terms of impaired performance and reduced productivity, and it may have been that way for years.

Much of the cost, both personal and corporate, is not yet calculated as tens of thousands of people, suffering stress-related illnesses, have not yet had those conditions recognized as such. Recognition of the vastness and variety of stress-related illness is beginning to surface, and awareness is increasing at an exponential rate in the field of medicine and reflected daily in the media. Once the parameters defining stress-related illness become well established, and more importantly, established in industrial law, an explosion of retroactive litigation may hit corporate society. In this legal battlefield, ignorance will not be an acceptable corporate defense.

Forward-thinking companies have established smoke-free workplace policies after recent landmark compensation decisions over secondhand smoke and its effect on people. We need to recognize, though, that issues like smoking and smoke-related illness are minimal in comparison to the overall question of stress in the workplace. Smoking is probably one of the simplest stress factors to identify and remedy.

The following is a statement of the Australian Community and Public Sector Union's policy on Work Stress. It was printed in the union newspaper *Our Voice* and, ominously in terms of my predictions, it was published in November 1990. Just about any organization could examine the list of stressors and working conditions in this policy statement and find, in their own situations, many elements that need addressing.

"The PSU recognizes:
1. That the presence of stressors in the work environment and the effect of these stressors are separate and equally important matters.
2. (a) The way work is organized can be a major stressor. Stressors include:
   • Repetitive work
   • Lack of promotional opportunities
   • Lack of job satisfaction
   • Lack of control over work...excessive pace
   • Poor management, rigid hierarchies, conflict with management or colleagues
   • Sexual harassment
   • Discrimination
   • Resource cutbacks
   • Insufficient staff
   • Excessive workload, overtime, irregular shifts
   • Job Security
   • Improper/inadequate training
   • Domestic responsibilities

   (b) Any problems with work conditions or environment can be a stressor:
   • Poor lighting

- Inadequate ventilation
- Heat and / or cold
- Noise
- Overcrowding
- Fumes, toxic chemicals, radiation
- Poor furniture
- Lack of protection from violent or aggressive clients

PSU rejects any notion of stress management which assumes stress to be a necessary part of work. It also rejects such stress management programs that treat stress as an individual problem to be dealt with by personal techniques and not as a hazard to be dealt with as an industrial issue.

The only stress management programs that are acceptable to PSU are those that recognize stress as an occupational and safety problem requiring collective action and greater control over work. Stress management techniques should only be used as part of the process to remove stressors and not simply cope with them. –David McKenna (National Industrial Officer)"

There is a revolution under way, heralded by such expressions as those of the PSU, by legislative reforms such as anti-discrimination and by concepts such as industrial democracy. Those companies that are proactive in the field of stress management will ride this revolution like a well-formed wave, reaping the real benefits it will bring, both to their corporate identities and performance, and to twenty-first century society as a whole. Those who delay or ignore the signs will be left floundering. Forward planning and appropriate action will bring a huge reward to companies that take the message to heart— not just in terms of avoiding costly litigation, but especially in increased productivity and a healthy bottom line for years to come.

## WHAT YOUR COMPANY CAN DO

1. Recognize the imperative and formally take action in *stated* company policy.

2. "Get with the program." An officer should be appointed with a status equivalent to manager to implement the policy. He or she should have:

(a) Access to all executive levels,
(b) Direct reporting and responsibility to the CEO and, crucially,
(c) Empowerment to staff and facilities.

Where the company is not large enough to support this level of investment in long-range planning, specialist external consultants may be employed. Initial expense in growing this corporate wing will be well rewarded when the enacted policy helps your company to soar above the stress management minefield.

3. Implement a program of education and training which covers the *entire* workforce. The recognition of the need for this has been confined to executive levels for too long. It's like concentrating all medical treatment on a headache when the headache is the result of infection flowing in your bloodstream to the brain from the big toe! The reality is that stress does not discriminate on the basis of hierarchy and it affects everyone (and their performance) from boardroom to office floor.

4. Initiate an urgent, professional review of workplace conditions and practices with a view to providing remedial strategies. Any examination that does not canvas the views and suggestions of every strata of the workforce will be inadequate, so comprehensive consultation with all employees is a prerequisite. This may well be the very first step after adjusting company policy.

## WHAT WORKS AND WHAT DOESN'T

Stress management programs often promise much but, in the long term, deliver little more than a healthy invoice for services rendered. There are a number of reasons for this.

First, the science is still young and is developing a response to urgent need. Management and personal development trainers and presenters, who may be specialists in their fields, are incorporating stress management into their packages and often deal with it as a component. It is, however, so important that it needs to be dealt with separately and specifically.

Human resources managers are daily presented with proposals for services in this field and it is extremely difficult for them to distinguish between gilt and gold. The high-flying "style over substance" programs inspire and uplift by virtue of the personal dynamism of the presenters (helped along by "special effects"), but invariably offer no long-term ongoing support, practical training, and education.

Approaches that depend heavily on attitudinal manipulations and on altering perceptions and habits have only short-lived success. The fixity of these attitudes, perceptions, and habits is the result of a lifetime's worth of inertia, not to be overcome in a weekend or a one-day seminar, at least not permanently.

Some management, when it has recognized the need to address stress, has presented programs (purchased at highly professional rates) and, in the aftermath, held the view that "now the problem has been solved." Stress management is not a dish to be served and eaten once or twice. It is an ongoing process, and has to be part of the daily diet.

For any form of stress management to be effective, it must address as many environmental factors and challenges in terms of working conditions as possible, and involve an ongoing pathway of training, education and support. Any program that doesn't offer this is a waste of funds. When engaging consultants, their value should be assessed on the basis of one simple question:

*Will the program lead to the establishment of an "in-house" structure that serves ongoing and future needs?*

# CHAPTER 2

## The Two Types of "Fight or Flight"

ONCE UPON A TIME, you walked along a jungle track. You suddenly stopped, absolutely still, and your nostrils flared as you sniffed the air. You were aware of your heart pounding loudly beneath your ribcage as you strained to hear the faintest sound.

On a branch above you, a jaguar crouched, also absolutely still, save for a slight twitch of the tip of its tail. Slowly, soundlessly, you moved your head slightly so that you could see, with your peripheral vision, the outline of the predator along the slim branch. Your grip tightened on your spear; your mouth was very dry.

To an onlooker, there was an explosion as the big cat launched itself; but to you, everything seemed to happen very slowly. You jumped aside and thrust upward with your spear—its fire-hardened tip entered the jaguar's belly and sunk deep. The spear was wrenched from your hands as the cat hit the ground and rolled, snarling, to one side. The shaft snapped and fell in the brush as the cat rolled and then stood looking briefly at you before launching itself at your face.

Instead of standing your ground and waiting to be hit—for you were a skilled warrior—you moved in and to the side, hardly noticing your shoulder sliced by the razor-sharp claws as the cat flailed in mid-air, misjudging its leap.

Even before the big cat hit the ground, you jumped on its back, encircled its throat from behind and with a mighty wrenching heave, brought your clasped hand and forearm snapping back. The sound of the neck breaking seemed to go deep inside you...and then you stood, legs and arms trembling, chest heaving as you sucked in huge gusts of air and looked down at the dead jaguar beneath you. You reached out your arms, threw your head back and roared a scream of triumph that echoed through the jungle. Brightly colored birds rose briefly in a noisy flurry from the tops of the trees, and then all was again silent.

You sank into the soft green jungle floor and lay there for some time. Slowly you became aware of the myriad sounds of life, large and small around you. You became aware also of the pain in your shoulder and the warm stickiness of the blood. You tried to move your arm and found it difficult—painful—and wondered at how the strength had poured into your muscles.

Once upon another time...you sit in a boardroom. There is a break in proceedings for five minutes and, when the meeting resumes, you will have to present the report that kept you at your desk until 3 A.M. that morning: the analysis and cash flow projection figures that you feel will spell the end—or at the very least the suspension—of the project you have been working on for the past three months. The persistent thought of the new government policy you heard on the radio, while you threaded your way through traffic, is all but drowned out by the unnaturally loud sound of the clock ticking. The policy will totally change the playing field and may negate all the negative conclusions of your report. But right now, your stomach feels queasy.

Around the huge table, which seems to stretch away forever, you are aware of the directors and other general managers. They are all engaged in conversation or reading from the notes in front of them. Your heart beats fast and loud beneath your ribcage and your temples throb painfully. You notice, with your peripheral vision, an assistant enter the room and move swiftly towards one of the managers, giving her a sheaf of papers. Your mouth is very dry, you breathe rapidly, and you become suddenly intensely aware of your own body odor mixed with the deodorant you hastily applied before leaving home.

The words *acute stress reaction* flash like a warning light in your mind. Instead of waiting in this limbo of anxiety for the meeting to reconvene, for you are a skilled warrior, you rise slowly and walk swiftly and purposefully to the washroom. Once inside you secure the door.

You press your palms against the sides of the cubicle and slowly apply pressure with your arms, while slowing and deepening your breathing, feeling your diaphragm moving deep down into your belly. You complete three steady, graduated pushes, then shake your arms loosely.

Gently you rotate your head in wide circles, in time with your breath, which is slower now, but not too deep. You feel the neck muscles releasing their tension. You cease that movement and then open your mouth as wide as you can, extending the tongue and tensing and contorting all the facial muscles. You glance at your watch and see that you still have two minutes, so you sit comfortably on the toilet and close your eyes.

You place the tip of your tongue against the roof of your mouth and begin to practice the "Centering Breath." After six rounds you rise and, keeping the calm, even flow of the Centering Breath, splash a little cold water on your face, briefly gargle with a little warm water, dry your hands and move with purpose to the boardroom. As you walk, the full implications of the new government policy start to sort themselves effortlessly in your mind and with each step you feel lighter and more filled with positive purpose.

As you enter the boardroom, faces turn toward you and you begin, "A funny thing happened to me on the way to the meeting this morning...."

## THE STRESS REACTION

The reaction to stress (or threat) is swift and comprehensive and lies entirely within the province of the body (although it may be initiated by the mind). The trigger mechanism is in a part of the brain that is not so linked to higher functions such as reasoning, but rather, concerned with survival.

This part of the brain, which includes an area called the *limbic system* and the *hypothalamus*, is often referred to as the "primitive brain." It responds with amazing speed to messages conveyed by the senses (and to mental perceptions) and can swiftly mobilize the body's resources, immediately prioritizing bodily systems in descending order of relevance to survival.

This "core preservation" system, the "fight or flight" mechanism, apparently has not evolved over recent millennia as much as the thinking, reasoning area of the brain, the *cerebral cortex*. The lightning reaction can still save you in life-threatening traffic or when you are walking alone late at night in a big city, but in modern society, the activation of the stress reaction is, for the most part, a totally inappropriate and disproportionate response.

## THE RELAXATION RESPONSE

It ought to be understood that there is a natural, innate counter mechanism to the stress reaction. It is the body's attempt to return to a state of balance and to redress the damage that can occur if the acute stage is prolonged, and is referred to as the Relaxation Response. It is a very real and ordered sequence of nerve transmissions, chemical, circulatory, respiratory, and muscular changes that must and—in acute, well-defined stress situations—does take place to bring all these activities back to "normal." (This will be addressed more completely in Chapter 5, "An Antidote for Stress.")

The wonderful thing about the Relaxation Response is that you can also activate it voluntarily; but—and it is this that makes all the difference in terms of how stress affects you—you have to learn to recognize the signs of stress. More importantly, you have to train yourself to be able to activate the Relaxation Response.

Going back to the scenario in the boardroom for a moment, imagine the process that may have ensued if you didn't recognize the stress reaction and didn't take any action to counter it. You are very tired and your mind is buzzing with all the figures you were juggling until 3 A.M. You and your team have been working very hard over the past three months on the project. If it is shelved or canceled, there is a real possibility that one or more of your researchers will lose their jobs. Jake, the latest addition to your staff, is the most vulnerable and he is struggling to pay hospital bills for his wife who is confined because of a difficult pregnancy. You really sympathize for his situation and you don't want to lose him as he is a brilliant and original researcher.

You find yourself sitting, swamped by a tide of associated thoughts and worries, and the new policy announced this morning is just a murmur beneath the general anxiety. Because of your mental tension, and your disappointment at arriving at the final analysis just before you switched off your desk lamp and tried to get a few hours' fitful sleep, you haven't been able to allow the full implications of the policy to surface properly.

Time zips by, and suddenly it is your turn to make the report. You begin by stumbling a bit on your introduction, as your tongue is dry and feels clumsy in the mouth. You try your best to convey the original inspiration for the project and give all the good reasons why it was begun in the first place, but you know there is no conviction in your voice and it is as if all your words are flat. You finally arrive, apologetically, at the conclusion and the final figures. Then, just as you are about to sit down, the government policy announcement surfaces in your mind and you ask, somewhat lamely, for another week to sort out the possibilities.

## STRESS MAY BE ACUTE OR CHRONIC

Acute stress is sudden in its onset and usually doesn't last for a long time. It may be brought about by a physical or a strong emotional situation (for example, the jaguar's attack). Chronic (that is, enduring for an extended period of time) stress is far more insidious.

Although the effect on the body is not as extreme as in acute stress, the imbalances that are created are maintained sometimes for years. Chronic stress is dangerous. It is dangerous because the process of habituation to the level of stimulus, the Relaxation Reaction, is not brought sufficiently into play and there is little opportunity for repair. Because we become used to operating at imperceptibly increasing stress levels, we don't see the need to do something about it. The stress reaction is prompted by either

external sensory information, or internal mental/emotional perceptions: for example, the passing of an ambulance with its siren
screaming (external), or a feeling of inadequacy or embarrassment
in speaking publicly (internal).

In neither scenario is the threat, registered by deep centers
within the physical brain, real or physical. However, the primitive
brain interprets the stimulus as being life-threatening and, accordingly, prompts the chain of chemical secretions which prepare us to
fight or fly: the "fight or flight mechanism." Primarily, the relationship of stress to illness is dependent on the inability to discharge or
utilize this altered blood chemistry.

## THE STRESS–DISEASE LINK

It is accepted in the medical profession that up to eighty percent of
illnesses have stress as a major component. If we look at the bodily
processes involved in the stress reaction, we can get a clear understanding of just how this "stress-to-disease" relationship operates.

Blood pressure rises quickly and dramatically. If maintained for
long periods, it can be a major contributor to cardiovascular disease:
heart attack, stroke, as well as other conditions. Blood clotting
potential also increases. Many so-called "heart attacks" are not simply (in spite of the popular view) the result of a mass of cholesterol
suddenly plugging up a coronary artery. They are, in fact, caused by
a spasm (like a cramp) of a vital heart vessel. Coronary artery spasm
is a direct result of stress, and can be sudden and devastating in a
heart that is otherwise perfectly healthy.

Blood gets drawn away from areas that the primitive brain swiftly
classifies as non-essential and is sent to the muscles of the arms and
legs to better enable you to fight or flee. The digestive system is particularly vulnerable. It doesn't really matter what's in your stomach
if you don't survive the stress event. The problem is that the primitive brain does not distinguish between real, life-threatening situations and those that may only threaten your job or self-image. This
mechanism can contribute to ulcers, colitis, candidiasis (a naturally
occuring yeast present in the intestines, held in check by the
immune system, but unchecked, can invade other areas of the body,

creating a condition assoicated with chronic fatigue syndrome), diarrhea, and constipation.

When blood supply to your skin surface is reduced, this interferes with the eliminative capacity of this organ and can increase susceptibility to rashes, psoriasis, and allergic reactions. Your lungs unconsciously try to take in more air. This can result in giddiness, fainting, and the so-called "panic attack," or hyperventilation, syndrome. This is a self-perpetuating condition, as the attack itself generates more anxiety.

Your immune system and the anti-inflammatory response are subdued, thereby increasing vulnerability to disease and infection. Blood cholesterol levels rise in response to stress. If this condition is maintained (effectively, a prolonged over-stimulus of the liver) then, not only is the vital function of this organ impaired, but the resultant changes in the walls of your blood vessels can present real problems. If this scenario is compounded by the regular over-consumption of alcohol to relieve the discomfort of stress, the liver is really under attack.

It is certain that modification of the stress reaction through physiological pathways can prevent the build-up of the stress chemicals in the system, but it is sensitivity and alertness to one's own inner climate that is crucial in developing the ability to use these pathways. In the next chapter we will look more closely at this inner climate, and help you tune in to your own "inner meteorologist."

# CHAPTER 3

# Your Inner Meteorologist

YOUR SENSITIVITY AND ALERTNESS to your own inner climate, both of which are crucial in developing stress mastering techniques, need to be awakened. This awakening is rarely spontaneous and, unfortunately, although it can and should be cultivated and taught as a basic life skill at the earliest stages of the education process, this is not the case.

We easily recognize the thunderstorm: the intense and sudden arousal we experience when there is an actual threat to life, and discharge of the body's stress chemicals is usually swift and comprehensive. However, it is living in a continual climate of "bad weather," the constant, unremitting, low-level stress of modern life that constitutes the real potential problem in terms of our performance and health.

## YOUR BODY IS THE BAROMETER

The difficulty lies in our acclimation; we become conditioned or habituated to the stressful situation and, in so doing, we don't perceive the need for discharging the accumulated chemicals on a regular, ongoing basis.

For example, you visit friends and, sitting down at the kitchen table for a cup of tea, you become aware of the incredibly intrusive noise produced by their old refrigerator. After the tea is poured and you have entered into conversation, you cease to be aware of the noise until it suddenly stops. At that point, you register that something has happened but you may not even realize that it is simply the silence, the stimulus being withdrawn. This is *habituation*.

If, as is inevitably the case in a progressively stressful work or home environment, the levels of stress chemicals have been gradually increasing or even maintained for an extended period, we tend to operate as if this is "normal." By this acceptance of continued "bad weather," we cease to register the effect it is having on our performance, health, and vitality.

First of all, we need to deal with the patterns of habituation that have become established in cumulative and chronic stress, and that means recognizing them. This recognition comes from first experiencing a state in which these patterns are not present (for example, the silence of the quiet refrigerator). Most people don't realize how far out of balance they have become unless they have the opportunity to consciously experience relaxation in the true sense of the word. (See Chapter 5: "An Antidote for Stress" for information on the Relaxation Response.) Once you have explored and enjoyed this experience, you have a new and essential life "yardstick" with which you can gauge your prevailing (I refrain from using the word "normal") biological levels of arousal.

Regardless of the effects cumulative, or chronic, stress may have on our mental and emotional state (and those effects can be profound and disturbing), the practical reality is that the dimension in which the impact of stress is primarily registered is the body. By learning and regularly practicing conscious and deep relaxation, we can increase awareness of and sensitivity to our bodily processes. We also begin to break the numbing patterns of habituation.

## CONSULTING YOUR INNER METEOROLOGIST

Once we have recognized stress as an ongoing factor in life, we can develop strategies and back-up systems to deal with it. If we don't, it is certain that we will suffer in terms of performance, poor health, and reduced quality of life.

Non-Specific Tension or NST (which means a specific cause for a high and maintained level of physical, mental and emotional tension has not been identified or isolated) is epidemic in our world. In reality, there is unlikely to be a specific, single cause as the condition is the result of cumulative, unmanaged (that is, unrecognized) stress.

With the generalized state of persistent arousal, which is symptomatic of contemporary life, comes an instinctive or unconscious tightening or habitual bracing against stress. This "tightening" is not confined to our musculature but is reflected in our body chemistry, brain function, attitudes, and mental and emotional state. Thus it affects our performance and relationships both at work and at home.

In the workplace, NST is most often evident in middle management, and is characterized by the "siege mentality." The manager suffering from this condition will be rigid and inflexible and will always attempt to operate "by the book" even though the book may be so far out of date that a whole new edition is required. Such people are usually hypersensitive to criticism and irritable. The condition impairs all their executive skills, including decision-making and the ability to have an overall and comprehensive view of a process or problem. This tension is both a symptom and a cause. The rigidity and inflexibility is an attempt at self-defense, but it negatively affects both personal interaction and performance, inevitably producing more stress, more tension.

If we only have one main programmed reaction to threat or challenge, whether it's getting flustered, angry, or feeling resentment towards the perceived source of the challenge, then withdrawal, a few extra Scotches or another glass of wine or whatever becomes the outlet. The programmed reaction is thwarted, and we experience frustration, and consequently more stress.

The degree of flexibility that you enjoy in your work and personal life is a reliable indicator of the effectiveness of your approach to dealing with stress. We can understand flexibility, not only in the sense of appropriate adaptation to challenges and change, but also in the simplest sense—the body. Are your neck and shoulder muscles free and mobile? Is your belly relaxed and comfortable? Are the muscles of your pelvic floor tight, or relaxed?

Flexibility under stress, together with freedom from the domination of your primitive brain center, has to be learned and cultivated. Your inner meteorologist arrives at conclusions about your developing climatic trends by one process: observation. The capacity to observe and monitor your own body must be developed, only then will you be able to intervene in a timely way to prevent the chronic build-up of stress and tension. You will have to get to know yourself.

## GETTING TO KNOW YOURSELF

What do you need to do to develop a deep and comprehensive relationship with anyone? You have to invest time with them. The more time you spend, and the more exclusive that time is of other, perhaps more distracting activities, the better the outcome.

In order to get to know yourself you have to spend the time. There are two levels of time investment: high-intensity exposure and frequent and repetitive short-term exposure.

### High-Intensity Exposure

The most intense time you can spend with yourself, to the exclusion of other distracting activities, is in the systematic and regular practice of the state of deep and conscious relaxation. This requires a commitment, but one that will provide measurable rewards in terms of your overall vitality and performance. You should allow a minimum period of twenty minutes daily.

Along with the familiarity you will develop with yourself on all levels during this practice will come the process of monitoring and observation and, most importantly, intervention throughout your day. (See the following exercise "The Six Events," and more in Chapter 15, "Stress Management Routines.")

### High-Frequency Exposure

By practicing "The Six Events" in your daily program, you will establish, however briefly, a systematic and positively habitual process of refocussing your energy (awareness) directed to whatever activity you're engaged in. At the specified moments throughout the day, you lift or accelerate your awareness into a more essential level. Whether you use the "Centering Breath," "Body Check," or simply become aware of your senses of sight or touch, you can bring yourself totally into the present moment.

A lot happens when you become totally present. There is a degree of instantaneous freedom from whatever may have been oppressing you mentally and emotionally. You are, for the moment, not at all involved in mental processes related to what has gone before or what may occur in the future. The short relief you provide yourself from repetitive, anxiety producing thought processes has, in itself, deep and positive implications in terms of your mental and emotional well-being.

Your body responds almost immediately to this shift in consciousness. It is as if you decide to "stroke" (that is, consciously encourage and shower with positivity) a close friend, or even your cat! The response is equally affirmative. Breathing slows and becomes more comprehensively efficient. Circulation to all parts of your body improves, especially to the brain. Blood pressure tends to normalize and the digestive processes improve. By lifting yourself into the present moment and by employing the following techniques, you activate the Relaxation Response.

So, this process of very intimate observation is not only one of monitoring your internal climate, but also one of active and therapeutic intervention of that climate.

CHOOSE UP TO SIX events or moments that regularly occur throughout your day, like taking your morning shower, turning the ignition of your car, pulling into the parking lot, going up in an elevator, having morning tea, eating lunch, buying your evening paper, traveling home, turning the key in your front door, checking your answering machine, etc.

**MASTERY SOLUTIONS IN PRACTICE:**

**The Six Events**

For example, let's look at your morning shower. Decide that you will be aware of each and every breath from the moment you enter the bathroom until you finish dressing. Don't try to control your rate of breathing, simply mentally become aware, "I know I'm breathing in—I know I'm breathing out."

Be sensitive to the flow of breath exclusively in your nostrils—do not breathe through your mouth. With each breath, try to move your awareness closer to the effortless flow in and out of your nostrils. Feel every millimeter of the progress of the air both in and out. Feel the difference between the warmer air leaving and the cooler air entering.

You can choose to do this from the time you turn the key in the car's ignition until you enter the freeway. Once you have read farther in this book, you will learn other techniques you can choose to apply at these times. The practices may vary at different times of the day, depending on your situation. The criterion that you should apply, as far as possible, is that the method should not interfere with the activity in which you are engaged, but preferably should enhance it.

This is painless reprogramming. The new is slipped in alongside the existing, unconsciously accepted habits of life. Done this way, the negative impact of change is defused and the benefits of the techniques can be felt immediately. The aim is to make the process as ordinary and natural as brushing your teeth.

Becoming present and activating the Relaxation Response for brief periods throughout your working day prevents the otherwise inexorable build-up of stress. You are counteracting the stress you are exposed to as it happens, not carrying an ever-increasing load. In the next section we'll look more closely at the factors that contribute to this stress build-up.

# CHAPTER 4

## The Playing Field

ON THE EVE OF THE millennium, we live in a rapidly changing, technology-oriented society. The impact of the separate elements, environmental degradation, the new demands of the workplace, and the rapidity of change itself that constitute this experience, let alone the sum of them, is deeply stressful. It is a challenging experience.

Success in dealing with the challenge lies in the process of adaptation and flexibility. Only in understanding each of the major stress elements can we develop strategies to deal with them. Often we are so caught up in the pace of life, swept along by its demands, we don't step back from it and have a good hard look at all of the aspects we really must deal with if we are to effectively enjoy it. In the face of what may seem to be a pessimistic analysis, it is important to remember that for every challenge there is an answer.

In this chapter, we not only give an overview of stress factors that you may not be consciously aware of, but also hope to alleviate anxiety that may arise from the analysis by suggesting ways of minimizing the impact of that stress.

## FORMS OF POLLUTION

The air we breathe, the water we drink and the food we eat are all contaminated to some degree. At the same time, we are establishing regulatory systems to, ultimately, reverse the contamination. The amount of pollution in our physical environment is the direct result of ignorance, although some more radical proponents of environmental purity and protection would have us believe that it is, at best, the result of capitalist greed or, at worst, some sinister plot by multinational corporations.

The ignorance is dispelled as it becomes obvious to companies and their shareholders that there is little point in posting huge profits at the expense of the environment if it results in no environment in which to enjoy that profit. What has been sadly lacking in our industrial and technological expansion is comprehensive, long-range planning for sustainability on all levels. The Environmental Impact Study, which is now a prerequisite for development, didn't exist thirty years ago!

### Air Pollution

For those who live and work in or near large cities and are constantly exposed to heavily polluted air, the effects of air pollution can be severe. Not only do the airborne pollutants cause respiratory disease and eye irritation, but many are also cumulatively toxic (i.e. they gradually build up in various organs and eventually impair the function of these organs.) Lead, although eliminated from gasoline in the U.S., is still very much a component of gasoline in many countries, and is a particularly noxious offender, leading to personality and attention disorders as it affects the brain itself.

Actually, one of the main ways by which these toxins find their way into our system is not by direct absorption through the lungs. The upper part of the respiratory tract, the nose and nasopharynx (the cavity behind the nose) is both coated with protective mucus and richly supplied with blood. Much of the contamination is trapped here and subsequently swallowed. It enters the digestive system, most damagingly at night (after a full day's exposure) where it enters the bloodstream.

Just as you wouldn't think twice about washing your hands after exposure to dirt, you need to become familiar with the practice of Neti. This simple, inexpensive and vastly therapeutic technique is not only immensely beneficial in preventing much of the negative effects of air pollution, but can also significantly reduce conditions such as sinusitis, recurrent head colds, and migraine headaches.

FOR THIS TECHNIQUE YOU should purchase a special Neti Pot. They are usually available through established yoga centers, or you may like to try a small teapot. Be sure that the end of the spout is smooth and will not damage or irritate the nostrils. Alternatively, much of the cleansing effect of Neti, if not most of the soothing, can be obtained by using a bowl.

> **MASTERY SOLUTIONS IN PRACTICE:**
>
> **Neti**

Add approximately one level teaspoon of salt to half a liter (500 milliliters) of warm water. A little practice will determine your comfortable concentration. Make sure it is around blood temperature, or approximately 98.6°F.

If you are using a bowl, dip one nostril in, while closing the other one with the finger, and suck the water through the nasal pharynx (the cavity behind your nose) into the mouth. You should proceed with this method slowly and gently to avoid inhaling the water. Spit the water out. I used this method for ten years before I was introduced to the special pots.

If you are using the Neti Pot, or a teapot, bend the head forward and turn it to the left, making sure that your mouth is open. Breathe through the mouth during the entire procedure. Introduce the nozzle of the container gently into the left nostril, so that the flared end forms a seal.

The water should flow easily into the nasopharynx (the cavity behind the nasal opening) and then out through the opposite nostril. If the water tends more to run down the throat, adjust either or both the angle of the head and the angle of the pot. Repeat the process from the right side.

Sometimes there is a minor blockage to the flow. This can often be cleared by closing the other nostril with the finger and gently sucking the water through the blocked nostril, spitting it out through the mouth. Once the blockage is cleared, proceed as normal.

Drainage: Immediately after practicing Neti, and especially if you are using the bowl method, it is crucial to drain any residual water from the area.

This is done by bending forward from the waist so that the head is hanging downward and exhaling rapidly several times through both nostrils. Sometimes you may clear copious amounts of mucus by closing one nostril and gently blowing through the open one.

You should blow gently; it is possible to force residual water into the opening of the Eustachian tube which leads to the ear. Raise and lower the head several times while continuing to bend forward at your waist, and repeat the process. (For a more complete description of Neti and its therapeutic applications, see Practice 7, page 165 "Neti.")

The use of living, green plants in the work and home environments is also a practical way of reducing air pollution.

Some of the air pollution that occurs, particularly in the work environment, is more subtle and also potentially very dangerous. Where there are many computer screens in use, the overall effect of this is to increase the concentration of positive ions in the atmosphere. The electrical charge of the particles is altered.

The effects of the buildup of positive ions were first detected during the U.S. space program. Astronauts suffered from a range of complaints, called "space sickness," including impaired concentration and digestive disorders, until the phenomenon was discovered and remedied.

In very simple terms, you feel energized but relaxed and vital in the forest, at the seaside or by a waterfall. This is largely due to the high concentration of negative ions. The opposite is the case in dry, dusty, or computer-prevalent conditions.

Air traffic controllers, in whose hands and concentrative abilities rests the safety of thousands of airline passengers, have approached this question out of absolute need by the installation of negative ion generators and effective filtration systems.

The research from the U.S. space program demonstrated that serious ionic imbalances can negatively affect the human organism at a microscopic level. Even the transport of molecules of nutrients through cellular walls depends on appropriate electrical charges.

It seems a pity that this information has not yet filtered through into mainstream business. If a company is striving for optimum performance in its employees and thereby optimum return on its investment in them, it is reasonable that the company make whatever adjustments may be necessary to the workplace. The installation of this sort of equipment can prove very cost effective by contributing to enhanced performance and productivity, and reduced illness.

I often make recommendations for the installation of large negative ion generator/filter equipment in open plan office situations, but if your company is unlikely to approve this, the purchase and use of a personal-scale negative ion generator that you place at your work station is an option. You may find that many of your colleagues gravitate to your area and the levels of your social and professional interaction at work may increase as they unconsciously tap into the invigorating negative ion field in your proximity!

## Water Pollution

The quality of tap water available in most large cities and residential developments is lamentable. It may be rendered pathogenically inert by chemical treatment but, in many cases, it is undrinkable, unless, of course, you happen to enjoy the taste of chlorine.

It is not just the quality of the water we drink that is in question, but also that in which we bathe. Very often this can exacerbate certain skin conditions such as eczema, dermatitis, and psoriasis.

If you live in a suburban house, it is worthwhile to consider the installation of both a rainwater tank for drinking purposes and a comprehensive in-line filtration system for your main water. With the rainwater tank option, it is important to have a primary diversion mechanism whereby the initial flow of water from the roof is diverted, as the water will contain much pollution. If you live in a city apartment, consider the possibility of purchasing distilled drinking water and also installing the in-line filter. Water is, however, much more than a simple combination of hydrogen and oxygen.

Distilled water may be pure, but it is basically lifeless. You can charge it by placing it in a crystal container in direct sunlight for thirty minutes before drinking. You will notice the difference!

In both residential situations there is an initial installation cost and ongoing maintenance, but this may be more than justifiable in terms of its benefits.

### Dietary Pollution

The effects of marketing pressures in food technology are now becoming more positively evident as we, the consumers, become better informed and educated. Where the power of food formulation was exclusively in the hands of the technologists, with a vast array of chemical additives to "improve" appearance, taste, shelf life, etc., the food industry is becoming more consumer-driven.

Many nervous, digestive, respiratory, and personality disorders have been attributed to pesticide and additive use in the production and formulation of food. Statements proclaiming the absence of these former additives now form a major part of product presentation, and the word "ORGANIC" has become a valuable mainstream endorsement rather than a reference to the obscure and purist gardening community.

But the pollution is still there. Additives are still being used, but there is a clear pathway through the junk-food minefield being illuminated. As the marketability of pure, fresh food increases, the cost benefits become more and more apparent. For very little extra outlay, it is now possible to largely avoid dietary pollution, even if you live in a large city. Simply avoid junk food and fast food. Buy organic and fresh wherever possible (it tastes better) and find an educated balance between what is optimum for your function and what you really enjoy. (For more information on this subject, see Chapter 9, "Food for Thought—and Action.")

### Noise Pollution

The effects of sound on the human organism are potentially vast and may be either destructive or therapeutic. Your individual response to this factor may, in part, be determined by your conditioned preferences (you may like heavy metal music) but, physiologically speaking, particular sound frequencies produce specific effects on your nervous system.

Experimentation with the effects of sound on plants and fish has demonstrated that some frequencies promote health and attract growth ( notably the more melodic and harmonious classical compositions) while others repel and discourage health and growth (such as the more cacophonic and disharmonious rock and pop music).

These lower organisms, compared to humans, have relatively unsophisticated nervous systems. Our response is amplified by the complexity and sensitivity of our nervous system. The overriding factor is our conscious mind.

We sometimes consciously seek out exposure to sounds that may be harmful to our physiological integrity and harmony in the belief that we are seeking "relaxation," but what we are in fact doing is looking for relief from what may be more powerful stressors in our life. The relief comes as a temporary distraction from those stressors.

Interestingly, in terms of occupational groups, classical music conductors have the highest levels of productive longevity, with many of them reaching peak performance in their late sixties. It may be inferred from this statistical fact that their longevity derives from prolonged exposure to positive sound patterns combined with a high degree of job satisfaction.

The levels of noise we are subjected to will vary according to our industry setting and our home environment. Much of it may appear beyond our control, but you can feel confident that the efficient use of healing sounds such as soothing "environmental" music and techniques such as the "Humming Bee" can greatly help to redress the damage that noise pollution can cause.

IN 1976, EXPERIMENTS WERE conducted in Madrid, Spain, to get an idea of the effect of self-generated sound on the human brain. The electrical activity of the brain was monitored in the subjects by electroencephalograph (EEG).

**MASTERY SOLUTIONS IN PRACTICE:**

**The Humming Bee**

A significant result was that the sound "Mmmmmm," when sustained for a period of time, produced identical patterns on the EEG

machine to those associated with deep, dreamless sleep. The subjects were very much awake and involved in an activity. Their subjective report was that they felt very calm, relaxed and centered.

The "Humming Bee" is a breathing technique that uses the
process of internally generated and specifically directed sound vibration to alleviate anxiety and to reduce cerebral tension (within the
brain itself).

Seated comfortably and with your eyes closed, inhale slowly. Don't
try to overfill your lungs, but rather, try to feel that the air is gently
and purposefully filling a hollow cylinder from your navel to your
throat. At the top of your inhalation, gently lower your chin towards
your chest and hold your breath (only for about three seconds).

Raise your head again, take a slight inward breath to open the
airway and simultaneously raise your hands, elbows out to your sides
to open your chest, and press your tragus (the small flap of cartilage
at the entrance) gently closed on both ears, using the tips of your
index fingers.

Using a controlled exhalation, make a humming sound. This can
be as subtle or as loud as your situation and discretion permit. Use
the whole exhalation to continue this sound: keep it as smooth and
uniform in pitch as you are able. (Find the pitch that feels most
comfortable to you.) Before you run completely out of breath, discontinue the sound and lower your hands to your lap.

At this point, when you are beginning the practice, it's fine to
take one comfortable normal breath and then begin again. However, the ideal is to establish a comfortable, controlled rhythm so
that the humming sounds are sequential. In order to do this, it is
important not to leave yourself short of breath at the end of the
exhalation and also not to inhale too fully. The essence of the technique is to establish the easy rhythm of breathing and a constant,
steady and unwavering sound.

Use the humming sound as a searchlight, moving its focus around
inside your head, left side, right side, top, front, back and center. As
you do this, your awareness should be within the physical brain
itself. Find the area in this space that you are spontaneously
attracted to and then focus the sound awareness there for the duration of the practice.

The soothing action of the sound produces changes in your brain chemistry and in your central nervous system. It can alleviate states of anger and anxiety, and it definitely reduces cerebral tension. It can also help greatly to relieve some types of headache. (For more information on this technique, see Practice 3, Brain Massage.)

## VISUAL POLLUTION IS VISUAL STRESS

Visual Pollution is not just a matter of tasteless billboards and ugly architecture. The degree to which the visual cortex of your brain is stressed is directly related to the light frequency and variety to which it is exposed.

If you drive to work for forty-five minutes at fifty miles per hour, you have already experienced considerable visual stress before you arrive along with the stress of a potentially life-threatening traffic stream. If you then sit down at your computer screen for several hours, you are continuing this situation.

The visual stress of the first situation involves the constant assimilation of input from a rapidly changing visual field—the highway. The second stress involves maintaining a fixed focal length and exposure to the light frequencies of your computer screen. Poor typists are actually blessed by having to keep looking at the keyboard and then back at the screen.

Here's an exercise: Look at your television screen or computer monitor and then shift your gaze to one side and relax your focus, so that you are registering the screen with relaxed peripheral vision only. You will notice that there is a high-frequency light vibration emanating from the screen.

This fluctuating vibration is there all the time, but you override it with your conscious mind, filtering it out for the end result, assimilating data. It is an unconscious irritation of the visual cortex and can severely interfere with your performance and sleep quality. The effect of prolonged exposure to excitation of this sort is, in a word, fatigue.

Here's another exercise to try. Simply decide not to watch television at all for a period of five days. You will be amazed at the difference in your overall vitality at the end of this period. Once you demonstrate the effects for yourself, you can make a reasonable choice about how much exposure you enjoy, based on your own experience. It is not unusual during this period to go through periods of extreme tiredness and changes in your sleeping pattern, as the brain seeks and uses the opportunity to restore itself.

The quality of visual exposure and resultant stress is increasing at a rapid rate. The impact of this is not confined to the visual cortex of the brain and the ocular system (the components of your eyes themselves). It also relates to the endocrine system (hormones) through the effects on the pineal and pituitary glands.

Rubbing your palms together to create heat, then gently pressing them against the closed eyes, together with eye exercises throughout the working day, can greatly help to balance the impact of visual pollution and stress. Significant moderation of television exposure and techniques like "Steady Gazing" (for more on this technique, see Practice 2) will also be of immense benefit.

## INSULATION FROM THE ELEMENTS

As we become more insulated (by our work and home environments, clothing and habits) from nature, we deprive ourselves of exposure to the healing and restorative power of natural elements. Here I refer to bioelectricity, not just our insulation from the beauties and aesthetic values of nature.

In ancient Greece, when the foundation for our modern Western medicine was being formed, there was a deep understanding of the importance of the elements of earth, water, air, and fire to the health of the human being. It was symbolically represented by the Hermetic staff, or the Staff of Aesculapius, which has become the symbol of modern medicine. This understanding seems submerged in the technological and pharmacological complexities of medicine today. In Chinese, Indian (Ayurvedic) and Tibetan medicine, the understanding has been preserved, and is alive and well.

Each of the elements has a therapeutic function and application in our lives, and although we won't enter into a detailed examination of them here, I make the following simplistic, but helpful, suggestions to incorporate them into your life experience.

Walk barefoot daily on the earth, on grass (you can remove your shoes during your lunch hour in a park), or at the beach. This is easily done if you live in Florida or California, but what if you are in the middle of a New York winter? There are alternatives. Every living tree is connected deep into the earth, even if its branches are bare of leaves and laden with snow. Make contact. I'm really not suggesting that you make tree hugging part of your daily routine—it doesn't have to be that obvious. Lean your back against the trunk, close your eyes, remove your gloves and place the palms of the hands against the bark. The backs of your hands will be kept warm against your coat. Focus on breathing mentally through the pores of the skin and feel an exchange of energy through the bark. As you breathe in, you are drawing earth's energy from deep in the ground, up through the roots, trunk and bark. Feel it flow up through both your arms, into the spinal cord and down to the base of the spine. As you breathe out, feel all tension drain from your being, through the tree and into the ground. This is the psychic version of "toxic waste disposal."

I had an encounter with a tree worth describing here. In 1968, my wife Angela and I had returned to Sydney, Australia, to stay with my mother after spending a year in New Orleans. We had been living a very intense and "pure" lifestyle, practicing six hours of yoga a day and eating only vegetarian food.

My mother, seriously Irish in her approach to nutrition, decided that we needed "feeding up." She also enjoyed the opportunity to "strut her stuff" for her daughter-in-law, and served bacon and eggs for breakfast, meatloaf for lunch and steak and potatoes for the evening meal. I discussed the radical change with Angela. We reasoned that polite acquiescence with my mother outweighed our dietary preferences and we decided that, as the situation was only temporary, we would simply accept and enjoy it as best we could.

After about ten days of this, I was suddenly struck down by a mysterious affliction. It began with excruciating pain in my toes and fingers and then swiftly spread through all the joints, including my spine. I couldn't walk properly and it was very painful even to sit or lie down.

I seriously felt I was dying and made preparations for my last days. Angela was wonderfully supportive, but we were both stunned by the intensity and suddenness of my illness. She drove me to a specialist clinic one morning for a comprehensive series of blood tests and other tests. Rather than return immediately to mother's house, I asked her to drive into the city and cruise around Moore Park, the Sydney equivalent of Central Park.

As we drove slowly through the park, I caught sight of a magnificent 100-year-old Morton Bay fig tree. I asked Angela to pull over. I got out of the car and made my way, painfully, over to the tree. It was huge and seemed to radiate calm and benevolence. Slowly, I removed my shoes and socks and leaned against the tree, with my face resting against the ancient bark and the palms of my hands flat against the trunk. I wasn't acting consciously, just responding to inner impulse.

The thoughts of soon leaving this physical world and being separated from my love rose like a wave and I found myself crying. The sadness engulfed me. Then I began to be aware of my contact with the tree. It was as if it had embraced me rather than the other way around. Quite suddenly I felt a surge of what I can only describe as infinite, soothing love and compassion. At that point I became aware that all the pain was being drawn out of my body, through the palms of my hands and the soles of my feet. It was an exquisite and exhilarating sensation. In moments I felt totally cleansed and free of all pain.

With a spring in my step and a huge grin on my face, I walked back to Angela, who was waiting by the car. When the results of the pathology tests came, it was pronounced that I had been suffering from an overwhelming build-up of uric acid crystals in all my joints. It wasn't very flattering to be told that another name for the condition was "gout," traditionally an affliction of the privileged nobility as a result of excess rich food and drink, but we immediately understood what had caused it. Medication was prescribed, but I never bothered with it as I'd already enjoyed my cure with a mighty dose of Morton Bay fig.

Drink water rather than "beverages" and use its bioelectrically cleansing effect by showering during your "Airlock" procedures at the end of the working day (see Chapter 12, page 100). In this situation, you're not showering to get physically clean, but rather to get psychically and electrically balanced.

Make "fire" the fire of regular physical activity (use the stairs rather than the elevator).

Use "air" in the energizing and balancing effects of the conscious breathing techniques to maintain equilibrium and suffuse you with energy.

## STRESS IN THE WORKPLACE

The stresses of the workplace are many and varied. Sometimes, no matter how ideal the employment may be, just the fact of having to go to work is stressful, particularly if this obligation conflicts with the demands and commitments of our personal life.

Design of work environments is an emerging science that will become more essential and refined as we seek to examine and understand the impact that stress has on employees in terms of their sustainability (i.e. performance, reduction of stress-related illness, etc.).

Previously considered to be less than essential elements in this design, aspects such as spatial interrelationships, lighting, color schemes, and background sounds are now all being taken into account for their effects on the individuals who comprise the workforce. The main criterion (with a longer term view of sustainability) does not have to be immediate and apparent efficiency.

If you "feel good" at your work station you will definitely perform better, so it makes sense for both you and the company to try to ensure that whatever can be done to create the feelings of well-being is done. The company has to get information and feedback from you about the effects of the work environment. How else will positive change occur?

The ways you deliver this information need to be examined to determine the most likely approach to get the result you need. Consult with your fellow workers first. Assess whether they have a similar response to the conditions, then use the means of expression you all agree on. Remember that "the bottom line" is as much affected by cost as by gross profit. The results of unmanaged stress can be costly!

Although the demands of some industrial settings are obviously such that it is difficult to totally apply this principle (e.g. the factory floor), there is always room for improvement and any improvement in the working environment will positively affect productivity, even if it is only by reducing absenteeism and stress-related illness.

WITH THE EXCEPTION OF a few rare instances, the provision of a dedicated physical space for the practice and use of stress management regimens is totally ignored by industry.

### MASTERY SOLUTIONS IN PRACTICE:

### The Washroom Retreat

More enlightened companies have made great progress in the provision of child care and in some cases, physical exercise facilities for their employees. However, the critical necessity for a "quiet zone" for use of those techniques that will allay anxiety, restore flagging concentration and realistically improve productivity and performance has not yet been generally recognized or accepted.

Though this may be lamentable, it is a reality we have to deal with in the present. However aggressively dedicated your company may be to "blind" efficiency, there is still one place where you are almost guaranteed a degree of quiet and privacy, and that is in a stall in the washroom.

In practical terms, it may well be that the toilets provide your best option for dealing with the day's stress when it manifests. The area may not lend itself to most of the techniques that require space and comfort, and may be especially inappropriate for deep breathing methods, but there is still much that you can do within its confines. It is often the only acceptable place you can retire to for periods of around five minutes. It can also help to avoid negative input from both the organization and fellow employees.

Choose the farthest stall from the washbasins and mirrors where conversation is most likely to occur. Once inside, with the door securely closed, put the seat down. This emphasizes the reason you have come there.

I know one executive whose company, in its infinite wisdom, opted for a vast, open-plan office layout, affording a total lack of personal privacy. At regular intervals throughout the day, she "goes into retreat" for exactly six minutes. Once inside the stall, she closes her eyes.

She then begins a very subtle form of the "Humming Bee," which she practices for exactly twenty-four rounds at the rate of four breaths per minute. She matches the pitch of her humming to the background sound of the building (air conditioning, etc.) and is secure in the knowledge that the very soft sound she produces is inaudible to others.

## YOUR CHAIR

An increasing amount of work is done while sitting. The impact of its effect on our health has been very much neglected.

The chair, which can and should be our friend, has become an enemy, responsible for insidious crimes against our health and vitality. It comes in many guises: the driver's seat in your automobile, the office chair and the many variations of domestic seating, the couch, the armchair, and so on.

In an unsupported sitting pose, the muscular and ligamental structures that maintain the lower spinal column are constantly and subtly exercised and strengthened. Your spinal posture is being regularly adjusted to the comfortable vertical. The whole spine, upper back and neck, not to mention the crucial nerve supply the health of internal organs and bodily systems depends on, benefit from this natural process.

However, when we sit supported in our chairs for thirty or forty hours a week, spend another twenty hours in our vehicles and flop into our armchairs for twenty or more hours of passive TV viewing, these supportive and protective structures are progressively weakened. The result can be impairment of adequate nerve supply to the digestive tract (constipation and poor absorption), and also to the sexual organs (impotence and menstrual problems).

The venous blood is impeded in its return journey to the heart and lungs. This can negatively affect blood pressure and interfere with heart and lung function.

Our hip, knee, and ankle joints are held immobile for long periods, and are rarely taken through their complete range of movement. This contributes in no small way to the onset of arthritic conditions in these areas.

When extra demand is placed on the muscular structures of the spine, especially the lower back, we are vulnerable to injury.

IF YOUR WORK IS largely sedentary, it can greatly help to get out of the chair at every opportunity. If you go to the washroom, consciously decide to use the facility on a different floor of your building, climbing the stairs to get there. Once you are securely locked in your stall, stand with fingers linked and palms downward. Slowly breathe in and simultaneously raise your straightened arms above your head while rising up onto the balls of your feet. At the top of the breath, stretch comprehensively, pushing the palms up towards the ceiling and feeling the muscular effort in your calves. Slowly exhale, bringing the arms and heels back to the floor in time with the outward breath. Relax. Repeat twice more.

> **MASTERY SOLUTIONS IN PRACTICE:**
>
> **In Your Chair**

While you are confined to the chair, consciously straighten the spine periodically. You can also consciously contract the muscles of your belly. Place both hands either on the arms of the chair or on your thighs.

Breathe out and, holding the breath outside for a few seconds, try to suck up the abdominal muscles by drawing your navel first back towards the spine, then, lifting your shoulders a little, up towards the chest. Relax the arms and the abdomen then breathe normally. Try to do this four or five times each hour. It only takes a few seconds and can have a wonderful effect on your energy levels and especially your digestion.

At home, you are free to sit in ways that can strengthen and maintain flexibility. Treat the floor as a friend and the chair as an enemy. Any of the cross-legged sitting positions and also the Thunderbolt Pose (see Practice 6, page 159) will help to keep the hips and ankles mobile and strengthen the spine.

One very important thing you can do at home to counteract the effects of sitting in a chair all day is to lie on the floor on your back for about five minutes with your legs raised slightly. Rest your legs on a chair or against the wall. Gently bend the feet and ankles back and forth, stretching the calf muscles. This uses gravity to help the blood flow back towards the heart, making its work easier, and helps prevent varicose veins.

## TOO MUCH...TOO LITTLE

The challenges you face at work may, although they generate stress, provide a good personal return in terms of satisfaction in your performance. This can hold true until the load becomes too great, causing you to feel that you are not coping. It also happens when there is insufficient challenge or stimulus, and you can feel undervalued and powerless. It is crucial to try to establish and maintain your own personal optimal levels of performance and satisfaction. Learn to communicate! Your superiors won't know your situation unless you advise them.

## HIERARCHIES

The previous rigidity of managerial hierarchy is now being forced to become more flexible and will be more so in the immediate future. Industrial and participatory democracy is becoming a widely accepted principle as its value becomes more recognized. Initially, because change is particularly stressful for the more autocratic and inflexible type of manager, innovations of this sort can be very unsettling. Once the benefits begin to flow from the synergy, they can find that their work actually becomes easier and the results are better.

## CAREER PATHWAYS AND WORK RELATIONSHIPS

The times are definitely changing for the better, with the effects of anti-discriminatory and affirmative action legislation and policy, but it is still a reality that many very competent and qualified women are still disadvantaged from progressing along their ideal career path. If you are in this position, the most important action you can take is to establish and maintain your stress management regimen, as the stress that is implicit in the impasse will negatively affect you if you don't deal with it.

You are expected to be dedicated, but with a change in the board of directors, new imperatives based on short-term results can mean you are suddenly out of a job! The level of insecurity and stress that poor management can cause is insidious and damaging to the whole structure of corporate health. Company loyalty is a two-way street.

Long-range planning for sustainability with more skilled, ethical and compassionate management is the only antidote for this disease. "Downsizing" and "corporate restructuring" are often not signs of vitality. The new broom "sweeping clean" or "surgical correction of corporate obesity" is often an admission and an indictment of poor management vision and planning.

If these policies must be enacted, for the survival of the company in the short term, their implementation must be accompanied by a frank and honest communication with the remaining staff to allay their anxiety.

The social and supportive aspects of relationships at work are also an integral aspect of dealing with stress. The interaction with colleagues can be dramatically improved by encouragement of social and recreational opportunities within the organization. In the new and progressive management climate, senior managers need not "keep their distance" on these occasions but can use them as ideal situations for the enhancement of an overall "team" perception.

## STRESS AS CHANGE

All change is stressful. We acquire patterns of response to situations that become unconscious and therefore effortless. When there is a change of any sort, be it negative or positive (and this may be largely a matter of individual perception), an adaptation is demanded. The adaptation requires effort and this represents discomfort, a disruption to our previously effortless and unconscious pattern of response.

## The Rate of Change

Any adaptation requires some time to assimilate the changed conditions and formulate appropriate responses, and time is a factor that seems to be in shorter and shorter supply.

As a society we are in great flux, constantly and rapidly adapting at many different levels simultaneously. The base of technology and knowledge broadens and the more vast it becomes, the faster the discoveries and changes that proceed from that knowledge become realities we all have to deal with. In one lifetime, in the twentieth century, we have gone through more changes than the previous ten generations.

The speed of the change itself is a major stress factor. We are, as a society, in a state of overload as we are only starting to become aware of the impact of the rate of change and are trying to develop comprehensive responses. To keep pace with it, and indeed, to enjoy it (for it is a wonderfully exciting time), it is absolutely essential that we have an effective regimen of stress management in place.

## HOME BASE

The more nurturing and supportive the home environment, the more prepared you will be to deal with all of the above. Work, and all the pressures you are subject to during that phase of your daily life, can severely damage the capacity of the home environment to provide this essential support, especially if you bring it home! (See Chapter 12, "Bringing It All Back Home.")

# CHAPTER 5

## An Antidote for Stress

THERE IS AN ANTIDOTE for stress, but it is a compound prescription, not a "single dose" answer. You will have to acknowledge and accept modifying your lifestyle to adapt to stress.

There are two levels of stress remedied by the antidote: the cumulative daily stress and then later in the chapter, the deeper levels: related to long-held perceptions and residues of emotional traumas that can undermine our performance and enjoyment of life. The antidote, most importantly, can also help us access our vast and dormant potential, providing energy, insight, and inspiration to deal with stress.

Before moving on to what I call the "prime ingredient" it is worthwhile to examine some of the lesser but important elements in your stress management prescription. The first of these is to establish and maintain a level of physical fitness by engaging in some regular activity that can give comprehensive exercise and appropriate discharge of stress chemistry. The subject of health and fitness is dealt with in greater detail in Chapter 6, "Holistic Health." Diet is also an important aspect (see Chapter 9, "Food for Thought—and Action").

Also, it is important to cultivate a positive outlook. This can only be done by practice. Negative thought patterns and perceptions are not confined to the mind. They produce an immediate and harmful alteration in your blood chemistry, which can produce a lower resistance to disease and impaired judgment.

## THE PRIME INGREDIENT: RELAXATION

We use the word *relaxation* to describe many activities that are in fact its antithesis! We speak of relaxing in front of the TV, having a cigarette to relax, relaxing at our favorite "watering hole" with alcohol, relaxing at the casino, relaxing at the movies, relaxing while playing cards or chess, relaxing with the latest spy novel, watching an exciting game of football, and the list goes on. These perceptions are a symptom of how little we understand the concept.

What is sought and achieved in the above situations is not truly relaxation, but rather, distraction and apparent and temporary relief from whatever may be the more potent stresses in our lives. Most of them provide a stimulus that can be exciting, and this stimulus can, cumulatively, be dangerous. It may veil a deeper illness, such as depression, or discontent, or a perception of social impotence.

Teenagers listening to heavy metal music, watching interminable cartoons, smoking marijuana, or gorging themselves on junk food are not relaxing. Statistically, this group has a high suicide rate.

Most of the activities that we categorize as entertainment are in fact stressful, but that is not to say that they are not enjoyable and, to some degree, beneficial.

Their benefits are directly related not only to the physical and environmental conditions, but particularly to the mental and emotional component of the activity. For example, what may be a beneficial, pleasantly stimulating game of golf can become a major stress event if you are playing with your managing director, or a valuable client whose account is due for renewal. If your level of identification with your hometown football team is deep and long-established, and they lose miserably, this too will affect you adversely.

### True Relaxation

The condition or state of relaxation that is the prime ingredient in your stress prescription is a process called the Relaxation Response, which may be initiated naturally and involuntarily by your body (to restore balance after a major stressful event) or consciously and voluntarily through the systematic practices of Deep Relaxation.

In Chapter 2, "The Two Types of 'Fight or Flight'" the process known as the Stress Reaction was described and the counter mechanism, the Relaxation Response, was also mentioned. Let's examine this process in more depth to fully understand what is meant by relaxation.

Your body and mind react and respond to stress through a framework called the autonomic nervous system. The word *autonomic* simply refers to the unconscious supervision of bodily functions and processes.

The autonomic nervous system has two branch functions. One is to stimulate, getting you out of the path of the car running the red light at the pedestrian crossing. This is the sympathetic nervous system. The second function is to restore balance and relax the body; it brings your heart rate back to normal when you find yourself safely back on the curb. This is the parasympathetic nervous system.

It is very encouraging to appreciate that, even a few short decades ago, medical science was of the firm opinion that the autonomic nervous system, and the processes it supervises, were beyond conscious control. Now, as we move into a new century, we know that we are able to consciously influence many of our bodily functions. We are learning and using valuable techniques, integrating them into our lives, and thereby growing and evolving to keep pace with the stresses, most of which we as a species have created for ourselves.

In the practice of conscious relaxation, the activity of the sympathetic nervous system decreases. Many positive changes take place in various bodily systems as a direct result of this. For example, within a few short minutes of entering a state of conscious relaxation, your metabolism begins to slow down. Blood pressure significantly lowers as the ongoing state of constriction of blood vessels maintained by the sympathetic nervous system is relieved and a more efficient blood flow is established.

Your rate of oxygen consumption can decrease by up to 20% and your heart rate is swiftly reduced during Conscious Relaxation. If you bear in mind that angina (the chest pain that is due to impairment of heart function or heart disease) is a direct result of insufficient oxygen being supplied to the heart muscles, the relationship is clear.

By comparison, it takes several hours (rather than minutes) for significant reduction in oxygen consumption to occur when you are sleeping, and the degree of reduction is usually only half that achieved in deep relaxation.

The state of conscious relaxation is the efficient use of energy. Your awareness is connected to the external world through your senses: eyes, ears, touch, smell and taste. You are looking out through the little balls of tissue and fluid at the visual field, presumably this text, and that process requires energy. For most of our waking life, we are externalized.

It's a bit like having a limited electricity supply, which is supplying light to lamps outside each window (the sense pathways) of your house, providing illumination for you to perceive what's happening outside. The supply is also connected to the internal lighting system but there's not enough power for both at the same time.

In the practice, you progressively and systematically withdraw the energy that is directed unconsciously into those sensory processes and make it available internally.

Conscious Relaxation is a process that leads to a deeply restorative condition. It establishes and maintains the hypnogogic or borderline state (for more on this subject, see Chapter 13), which permits efficient discharge of stress chemistry, and thereby relieves cumulative muscular tension.

This state, which amounts to turning off the outside lights, can then be a platform from which you can proceed to intimately and efficiently explore yourself on a physical, as well as mental, level. When the internal climate is positively adjusted and this platform established, you are then able to concentrate with an efficiency that may astound you.

## CONCENTRATION

The concentration potential you make available is the gateway to deeper levels of your being. Once you establish the borderline state, you can then start to use deeper techniques such as Inner Silence and Visualization.

Normally, when we try to concentrate, we have limited success depending on many variables, such as the environment and our mental and emotional state at the time. We are usually able to maintain concentration for a period, but then get unwittingly dragged down the winding corridors of associative thought (where one thought leads to another, and so on) and we end up thinking about something totally different from our initial focus. We have not been trained to think!

## ACHIEVING INNER SILENCE

Inner Silence is a systematic way of training yourself to think. It can hone your thought processes to a razor-sharp edge, adjust your perceptions of both yourself and others and liberate you from the domination of anxiety, worry, and obsessive, repetitive thinking.

By clearly defined stages you become aware of the workings of your own mind, gradually developing the faculty of thought direction and control. You not only observe reactions and thought processes, but also progressively open the gateway to your own subconscious. The intimacy of your own self-exploration and understanding is such that you truly become "friends with yourself." In a gentle, friendly and objective way, you become progressively capable of releasing and defusing traumatic and deeply stressful experiences and memories.

The technique involves establishing and maintaining a state where no thought comes. This is not an emptiness or "mental vacuum," but an ongoing, intensely aware and totally present condition of focused concentration.

This extraordinary state of being improves memory, restores balance to the personality and can provide superb mental and perceptive clarity and accuracy. After the death of my wife Angela, this was the single most effective technique I used. I was able to move through the grieving process swiftly, and come not only to a point of acceptance, but to one of joyous understanding.

Without waxing too lyrical about human potential, it's necessary to give a viewpoint here that is both optimistic and inspirational. If you persevere long enough in the state of one-pointed concentration, you create the possibility for accessing potentially dormant areas of your brain. It is said that we operate on only twenty percent of our brain power and, to carry the light and power analogy a bit further, it is as if the remaining eighty percent of our brain is a sleeping city.

In order to turn on the lights and empower the city, we must make a connection with a power source much greater than the limited supply we initially used. There is a vast reservoir of bioelectrical energy you can access. Throughout history there have been many people who were able to tap into this energy: inspired scientists, artists, musicians, and humanitarians.

This energy is called "chi" in the Oriental martial arts, and in the science of yoga it is called "Maha Shakti" or "the great energy." When you do connect with it, all the lights will come on in the sleeping city of your brain. But, before you can throw the switch, a new line has to be installed that is capable of safely carrying the high voltage. In other words, the body and the brain have to be properly prepared.

There are many disciplines in many different cultures that aim at the systematic preparation for, and ultimate utilization of, this energy. It is unfortunate that, until recently, they have been scientifically ignored due to cultural and social prejudices. It has also been difficult to extricate the actual, valuable techniques from the cultural myth, superstition, and religions into which they have been woven.

That is changing. East is meeting West in an unprecedented exchange. We are examining these techniques pragmatically and analytically, and then adapting and integrating them into our culture. As a practicing Yogi for thirty years, I have drawn greatly on the vast body of experiential knowledge contained in this science for much of my approach to stress management.

When you recognize the absolute imperative to deal effectively with stress and begin to integrate these techniques into your life, you will grow from challenge to challenge, raising your performance levels, and ultimately, your enjoyment.

From a human evolutionary point of view, it should be understood that the stresses that we as a species are subject to constitute the impetus to evolve. Stress is not bad. It is an essential stimulus, prodding us to change and grow to reach our maximum potentials.

SIT COMFORTABLY IN A chair or on a cushion, with your back supported. Close your eyes and become aware of your natural breath. Don't try to deepen or slow it down, just observe it. With each breath, mentally repeat, "I know I'm breathing in, I know I'm breathing out." Do not control it.

> **MASTERY SOLUTIONS IN PRACTICE:**
>
> **Inner Silence**

Focus your awareness of the flow of the air exclusively in your nostrils. Feel the difference between the cooler air entering with inhalation and the warmer air leaving with exhalation. With each breath, move your awareness closer and closer to this natural tidal flow, trying to feel every tiny millimeter of the movement of the air in the nasal passage, both in and out. Keep mentally repeating, " I know I'm breathing in, I know I'm breathing out."

Now choose a number and count backwards to zero. The number you choose depends only on the time you have available. For purposes of this exercise, let's start with 30. "I know I'm breathing in, I know I'm breathing out—30. I know I'm breathing in, I know I'm breathing out—29, and so on back to zero. This should increase the quality of your sensitivity and awareness with each breath. Treat each breath as a separate adventure, to be explored and experienced.

When you finally reach zero, imagine that now you are breathing, both in and out, through every pore in the whole surface of your skin—over the whole body. As you inhale, imagine your breath entering your body through every pore as a golden light, filling the entire space within the envelope of your skin with golden radiance. Also imagine a feeling of expansion with inhalation, imagining your whole body becoming so light that if a breeze came, it would drift like a balloon on a string.

As you exhale, create a feeling of letting go. Feel that you have the power to focus your awareness on your breath leaving through the pores of the skin in any specific body part you choose. Select areas you may have experienced tension and feel that tension leaving with the outward breath. Play with this visualization for a little while.

Now choose a thought for yourself. It may be about anything at all. Be aware: *I am observing this thought.* Develop the thought. It may be a word sequence, an idea, or a picture, but don't allow any other unconnected thought to intrude. Maintain this theme for a while, simultaneously being aware: *I have created this thought for myself to observe. I am a witness.*

Now, start to bring yourself back. Become aware of your body's weight, its density and solidity. Feel the whole body as one unit, a complete whole. Mentally repeat "Whole Body" several times and feel it all in the same instant. Slowly open your eyes just enough to let a little light in—but don't focus them. Stay like this for a few seconds, being generally aware of the act of "seeing." Then release the position and have a good stretch. (For more information on Inner Silence, see Practice 10, page 185.)

# Chapter 6

# Holistic Health

HEALTH AND STRESS ARE intimately connected. Your capacity to deal with stress will be largely determined by your state of health and your health is directly related to the effectiveness of your mastery over stress.

In Western orthodox medicine the focus, until recently, has been on disease rather than on health. Truly healthy people were not examined to determine the standards of "normality" but rather, statistical averages (with the vast majority functioning well below optimum) were used.

The body was regarded from a more or less mechanical viewpoint. Now it is well understood that our mental and emotional states directly affect our bodily function, mainly through the direct interaction of hormonal and chemical levels.

An acceptable definition of health, mental and emotional as well as physical, is not simply the absence of disease. True, holistic health is an abundance, an overflowing of vitality and energy. This abundance should apply to body, mind, and spirit.

## SENSIBLE MEDICINE

I have the highest regard for modern Western medicine. Its diagnostic system is unsurpassed and its capacity to treat life-threatening disease effectively increases daily. However, until recently, its approach has been curative rather than preventive. There is really no choice to be made. The two approaches are not mutually exclusive. A combination of both is a much more rational approach.

The alternatives, which include acupuncture, naturopathy, osteopathy, chiropractic, homeopathy and herbalism, each have much to offer, and, apart from their specific therapeutic applications, can approach health with a view toward education and illness, toward prevention.

There are pitfalls for patients and practitioners in both fields, however, so negotiating the "health minefield" safely is a realistic and pragmatic attitude. You need complete confidence in the professional you choose to help you through any illness, so don't be afraid to ask questions. Be guided by your own assessment of the therapists. Do they appear to be healthy themselves? This is a fair yardstick to apply.

Be a pragmatist and avoid over-identification with any healing practice. If your house is on fire, you call the fire department and you don't worry too much if the firefighters trample on the flower beds as long as they save the house. If you have illness or infection, which may be potentially serious, especially in areas such as eyes and ears, don't hesitate to consult a properly qualified medical practitioner. You can always replant the flower beds or, in the case of dealing with infection by using appropriate antibiotics, you can balance whatever the side effects of these may be after the crisis has passed by using naturopathic methods.

## THE POWER OF THE IMMUNE SYSTEM

Your immune system is the immigration control center of your personal territory. This territory is under constant threat of alien invasion in the form of pathogenic bacteria, viruses, etc. and your security forces check the "credentials" of all new arrivals. If they don't have the correct "identification," they are dealt with quite ruthlessly.

If you remember that every time you breathe in, or put your finger to your lips, you transfer thousands of potentially harmful organisms into your system, the importance of the immune response becomes clear.

The immune system not only stands guard at the gateways of the body, it also performs quality control in the process of cell replication. Old cells are constantly being replaced by new ones at the rate of millions a day. Wherever there is large-scale production of this sort, there will always be rejects—the occasional distorted, poorly programmed or aggressive reproductive cell will be made. The immune system destroys all those that don't meet the body's strict standards for the maintenance of its integrity.

All goes well on both fronts until, and unless, the security forces are taxed beyond their endurance. Where there is constant and unremitting stress, the same systems that constitute the immune response are constantly stimulated and prodded. It's reasonable that their performance flags as they become less alert. If an unwelcome alien gets past their screen, ducks down a corridor into a warm, dark, moist corner and starts to breed, the result may be influenza. If an aggressive reproductive cell is manufactured and slips past the quality control mechanism, the result may be cancer.

There was a very dramatic case in the mid-seventies in America where a kidney transplant recipient received a donor organ that contained, unknown to the transplant team, a cancerous nodule. Because the patient's immune system had to be medically suppressed to avoid rejection of the transplanted organ, the cancer in the donor kidney grew at a phenomenal rate and spread rapidly, invading his whole body. Once doctors realized what had happened, the immune suppressant medication was withdrawn, and within twenty-four hours the cancer had completely disappeared from the patient's body, and had withdrawn to the donor organ.

The kidney was subsequently rejected by his body, but the amazing sequence of events, from a cancer-free state to being riddled with cancer and back to a cancer-free state, all within a three-to-four-day period, was a powerful demonstration of the immune system.

Genetic predisposition aside, the maintenance of your body and mind in a balanced state will go a long way to preventing the occurrence of illness or disease.

Body and mind are virtually interdependent, and whether we call it the bodymind or the mindbody depends on the direction from which we approach our examination.

## BODY HEALTH AND FITNESS

One of the vital components of health is fitness. Fitness implies much more than just a freely mobile skeleton with strong and supple musculature. It also means a healthy cardiovascular and respiratory system, hormonal equilibrium, efficient digestive system, balanced nervous system, and a highly alert and functional immune system. The primary pathway to this fitness is through an enjoyable and efficient discipline of exercise.

### Exercise Choices

Unless your occupation provides you with natural opportunities for exercise (such as a professional sports person), it is vital that regular and comprehensive exercise be incorporated in your daily regimen. Regularity means establishing a pattern of frequency that can provide adequate discharge of stress chemistry and maintain a good level of fitness.

This may mean that you join your local gym and attend at least three days per week. The best approach, if this is your chosen expression, is a supervised and monitored program of "circuit" training, where all the major muscle groups are proportionately worked and toned, as well as the joints. Joint articulation is often inadequately dealt with in some circuits, but is addressed more comprehensively in the aerobic-style workout. You may wish to incorporate a moderate session of joint articulation into your routine.

The gym has some advantages over other plans. First of all, it requires that you actually remove yourself from your accustomed environment, and the change of venue itself can be refreshing and motivating. The available equipment is also specific and inexpensive to use.

However, in a busy lifestyle, it is often difficult to maintain a schedule with regularity as gym attendance usually depends on some travel, which itself can take valuable time. It is often the case that, if for any reason you are prevented from getting to the gym by events in your personal or work life, the pattern of attendance is broken and may be difficult to restore. One drawback of gym work is that its approach can be very one-dimensional.

Walking can be a wonderful way of establishing fitness and it can address other aspects of stress management at the same time. It helps to establish healthy cardiovascular performance, and can also help prevent varicose veins for those with largely sedentary lifestyles.

Your walks can be planned to take you along different routes, and you can explore parks, nature reserves, and beaches. It can be a very enjoyable, low impact routine that is refreshing and efficient (provided you walk approximately three miles daily). But walking is subject to weather and, again, if the pattern is broken it can be difficult to restore.

Competitive sport can also provide many benefits, including fitness and great personal satisfaction. There is often considerable opportunity for the discharge of accumulated stress chemicals and to vent emotional frustrations and tensions, too. The one aspect of this discipline which needs to be appreciated and balanced in terms of your enjoyment is, especially as you get older, the potential for injury.

The best recommendation I can make in terms of establishing comprehensive fitness is to learn and practice a combination of yoga techniques specifically tailored to your personal requirements. Initially this might mean attending classes for a time to master the basics, then eventually in consultation with your instructor, develop a personal program. When you arrive at a level of moderate proficiency, and it's no longer necessary for you to attend (unless you really enjoy the class situation), you can effectively practice at home.

There are advantages to choosing yoga as your path to fitness. It doesn't require any special venue or equipment, and once you become an independent practitioner it can be done at home, and will cost nothing. It is also very low impact and addresses you on the deeper levels of the nervous system and hormonal equilibrium, as well as dealing with the other aspects of fitness.

There are many different approaches to yoga instruction and, as with some gyms, some of these are less than comprehensive. When making inquiries about a particular yoga school, ask the teacher or receptionist what happens during the class period. Ideally the class composition should be around forty-five minutes to one hour of postures, and the remaining time should be devoted to breathing techniques and conscious relaxation.

Whatever approach you take to the issue of exercise, one of the most important criteria is: Does it make you feel good and do you enjoy it? This enters into the realm of the mind, and it is important. If you impose a severe discipline on yourself with the intellectual approach of "I must do this because it is good for me," even though deep inside you are screaming "No, no, I really don't like this—it hurts!" the cold hard reality is that you will not persevere with it. Sooner or later you will find some perfectly good reason to stop.

THIS IS A COMPREHENSIVE form of potentially aerobic exercise that positively affects not only the major muscles, joints and spinal column, but also the internal organs. It requires no special equipment and, for best results, should be performed in the early morning after bathing, although it may be used at any time of day to restore flagging energy and mental vitality.

**MASTERY SOLUTIONS IN PRACTICE:**

**Sun Salutation**

It consists of a flowing movement, synchronized with the breath, through a series of twelve positions. One complete round consists of two repetitions of the sequence.

> **Position 1:** Stand for a few moments, feet together and palms of the hands gently touching at the chest. Close the eyes and relax the whole body. Breathe normally for a while, then exhale fully.

> **Position 2:** As you inhale, separate the palms, extend the arms out in front of the body and, in time with the inhalation,

raise them above the head. At the top of the movement and the breath, the head and upper back are inclined slightly backward.

**Position 3:** Slowly exhale and, maintaining the relationship of extended arms and head to the trunk, bend forward from the waist until, at the end of the exhalation, your hands are as close as comfortable to the floor while keeping the legs straight.

**Position 4:** As you inhale, while bending the left knee, lower the pelvis and stretch the right leg back, toes and knee in contact with the floor. At the same time the head is inclined backward, the spine extended and the gaze is directed at the ceiling. Weight is supported on the hands, left foot and the right knee and toes.

**Position 5:** Taking the weight mainly on the hands and right foot, exhale while raising the buttocks in the air, straightening and extending the left leg back so that the foot comes to rest alongside the right. Allow the head to hang. Heels are as close to the floor as the straightened legs will permit. Having arrived at this position at the end of the exhalation, keep the breath outside for a few moments as you move into Position 6.

**Position 6:** Keeping the breath outside for a few moments, lower the body to the floor by bending the knees and elbows. Chin, chest, palms, knees and toes are in contact with the floor, while the buttocks are kept raised so that the lower belly and pubic bone are suspended.

**Position 7:** Exhale just a little more, to open the airway, then, as you slowly inhale, raise the head and upper back, straightening the arms and making sure the pubic bone is in contact with the floor. Relax the lower back in this position.

**Position 8:** Exhale, straightening the arms and legs, while raising the buttocks again as you did in Position 5.

**Position 9:** Taking the weight on the hands, left knee and toes, slowly inhale as you bend the right knee, bringing the right foot in one fluid movement to come to rest between your hands. Arch the head and torso backward.

**Position 10:** Taking the weight on the right leg and hands, exhale as you release the left leg and bring the foot alongside the right foot. Straighten the legs and allow the hands to be as close to the floor as comfortable. this is the same as for Position 3.

**Position 11:** As you slowly inhale, bring the extended arms, trunk and head up to a repetition of Position 2. Lead the movement with the head, bringing the spine to the raised position vertebra by vertebra.

**Position 12:** Exhale as you come into this final position, which is exactly the same as Position 1.

These twelve positions constitute one half round. To complete a round, repeat the movements as above except that in Position 4 the left leg is extended back and in Position 9 the left foot is placed between the hands.

## MENTAL REST

Now that you have settled on a form of exercise that will suit you and provide the basis for physical fitness, you need also to develop an approach that will give you a balance of mental stimulus, enjoyment, and rest. You probably naturally gravitate easily toward some stimulus and enjoyment. Now you must turn to the issue of mental rest.

In Chapter 5, "An Antidote for Stress," a brief description of the process and benefits of the "Inner Silence" was given. This specific technique can provide, more efficiently than sleep, a very deep quality of mental rest. At the same time you become gradually more proficient at something we believe we can all do, (but something we have never been trained to do effectively), and that is thinking!

Whenever you experience a worrying or anxious thought, there is an immediate and corresponding physiochemical reflection of that thought in your body. If the thought processes are repetitive or obsessive, this can be an exhausting and oppressive situation. If such processes are sustained, they can deplete the immune system and make you vulnerable to disease or illness. In short, negative thinking can make you sick.

Learn to suspend thought. The most complete approach to developing this capacity is contained in the "Inner Silence" method. As well as exploring this technique there are other things you can do such as bringing yourself totally into the present moment by focusing on either a combination of the senses or just one sense (such as sight, touch or hearing) in isolation. If you establish and maintain an attitude of being totally present to each stimulus—even for a few moments—it can be very therapeutic.

When you narrow your field of awareness, through your senses, and bring yourself totally into the present moment, for that period there is no stress—just the activity of being aware.

### An Exercise

As you sit and read these words, become aware of the components of the experience of reading. First, there is the visual field: the page and the text. Second, there is the medium of perception of that field, your eyes themselves: the little balls of muscle, tissue and fluid through which you are looking out at the visual field. Third, there is YOU, your awareness or consciousness, who is looking out through the eyes at the page.

Rotate your awareness and sensitivity among these three components of the experience, letting it rest briefly on each in turn. Visual field; my eyes (feel, sense, become aware of, the eyes themselves); I who am looking out through the eyes (call it "Self"). Go on moving your awareness for a few seconds: Visual field—eyes—self.

### Another Exercise

Become aware of your sense of touch. Take your awareness on a swift journey around your body and locate the exact meeting points of the body with its environment. Start at the floor, feel your feet in your shoes, the contact with the seat, feel the contact of your clothing with the skin, your fingers holding the book, points where the body contacts itself (upper lip against lower lip, the tongue in the mouth, inside of the upper arms contacting the sides, the armpits).

Move very swiftly, just like a spark jumping from one point of contact to the next, and go around the whole body in this exploration several times.

If your mind is immersed in worry, depression, or anxiety, it needs, first of all, to be brought out of that mode before you can effectively or rationally resolve whatever may be the cause of your negative state. It is next to impossible to resolve matters or to think clearly, with sufficiently wide perspective, while you are in the thrall of depression or anxiety. The most efficient way of removing yourself from the influence and oppression of your mind is to shift the focus to the physical. The old advice "take a cold shower" has a firm basis in practicality.

Another technique that can be effectively used to suspend unproductive or negative thinking is the breathing technique of "Brain Massage," described in detail in Practice 3. This technique consists of short, sharp exhalations through the nostrils, followed by a brief suspension of the breath. It invigorates the brain, bringing well-oxygenated blood, and interrupts the pattern of repetitive, obsessive thought.

It is essential, if you want to be a healthy and whole person, to appreciate that exploring and understanding your own mental processes—and developing a basically friendly relationship with your mind—is just as important, if not more important, than making sure your diet and exercise needs are met.

## THE FOCUS OF SPIRIT

There is more to life than "birth, death, and taxes." To be truly healthy, it is crucial to find your own spiritual focus, and to make that the platform from which your life and activities proceed.

My approach to spirituality (which I perceive as the animating and unifying energy in my life) is through the enhancement of my conscious awareness.

Whether your spirituality is focused in organized religion, or involves a sense of intimate connection with nature, it needs to be a living and vitalizing source of energy and inspiration in your life.

In order for your spiritual expression to assume its rightful place, and thereby to provide its inherent wealth of benefits, it must be practiced.

Plan to incorporate this practice, whether it is reminding yourself from time to time as you go about your daily tasks or visiting the cathedral, synagogue, mosque or beach, on your way to or from work. At its simplest level of value, your regular spiritual practice can provide a series of positive moments during which you reorient yourself. Those moments allow a deeper and wider view of priorities that can otherwise be submerged and lost in the pace of life.

# CHAPTER 7

# Pathways of the Breath

FOR YOUR BRAIN, YOUR own bio-computer, to function at optimum level, fuel or power is required. That fuel is air. Without it the computer shuts down and quickly dies. The socket through which you are plugged into this vital power grid is your nose.

For the power, in its raw state as air, to be available to your brain, it is first transformed, and then transported, in a specific conductive system—your bloodstream. In its raw, gaseous state, this power must be changed into a liquid before it can be carried to your brain, and simultaneously to your whole body, which is monitored and directed by your brain.

When this gaseous exchange occurs in the walls of the tiny lung sacs, called *alveoli*, there is an optimum temperature and humidity for the power transformation to take place. The nose and the passage and cavity behind it, the nasal pharynx, are absolutely vital for establishing these ideal conditions.

The nose and nasal pharynx form your personal air conditioner. Large airborne impurities are filtered through the hairs, and smaller particles are trapped on the mucous lining of the passage. The entire area is richly supplied with blood in thousands of tiny vessels called capillaries. The outside air temperature can be below freezing as it enters the nose, but this very efficient conditioning system can raise that temperature to body heat over a distance of just twenty-five centimeters.

It's been said that as humans have evolved, our "higher" functions have become more developed and specialized, but our sense of smell has become less discriminate. This is completely untrue. Our sense of smell is as acute as it ever was. It provides us with an "early warning" system but, as civilized and sophisticated beings, we tend largely to override this information when it doesn't agree with our mental analysis of a situation.

For example, you are invited to dinner by a couple you met in friendly circumstances. Supper is at seven o'clock, and you turn up on their doorstep with a bottle of chardonnay in hand and ring the doorbell. The door opens after a small delay and your host and hostess greet you, and seem happy to see you. They smile and welcome you inside.

You take one step inside and immediately feel uncomfortable. You feel a little tightening inside and you know something is not quite right.

Ten minutes before you arrived, your friends had a heated argument, an intense domestic quarrel over suspected infidelities. Then, two minutes before you arrived, they suddenly remembered your arrival, and with considerable effort, dragged themselves out of the fight. They splashed some cold water on their faces and tried to prepare themselves as best they could. No matter how much they smiled, you knew something was wrong and if asked, you would probably say that there was tension "in the air." You can bet it was in the air!

When we feel angry or fearful, very subtle chemicals are emitted by our bodies. They are called pheromones. They enter the atmosphere in incredibly small concentrations, but your sense of smell detects them, recognizes the fear chemicals or the anger chemicals, and sends the message straight to the primitive brain centers where your own "fight or flight" mechanism is initiated.

Colloquialisms such as "tension in the air," "gut feeling," and "I smell a rat" all have a physiological basis. When your "fight or flight" reaction is prompted, blood is withdrawn from the digestive organs as the defensive primitive brain directs it into the large muscles of your thighs and arms. This can produce varying degrees of unease or discomfort in your stomach and belly. Conversely, when the parasympathetic nervous system takes over and you experience relaxation, the blood flows back to this area creating warmth and comfort.

It is absolutely essential to cultivate the automatic habit of breathing through the nose if you want to perform at optimum level.

Your breathing pattern accurately reflects your prevailing mental and emotional climate. How you think and feel is shown by how you spontaneously breathe. There are two basic and distinct spontaneous breath patterns that are related to, and are symptomatic of, opposite states of being. It is an incontrovertible fact that neither of these breath patterns can co-exist very long within its contrary mental or emotional climate. It is absolutely impossible to be relaxed, calm and centered and breathing spontaneously in a fast, ragged, and shallow breath pattern. Conversely, you cannot be angry, anxious, tense, or frightened and breathe spontaneously in the slow, deep, and even pattern.

I have used the word *spontaneously* to emphasize how breathing naturally reflects your state of mind—that is, when there is no controlling mechanism in place. If you can consciously initiate the opposite breathing pattern, the mode you are in must and will change.

It doesn't happen immediately. It takes some time. Just how much time depends on your familiarity with the process and the efficiency with which you approach it. Of course, you must first be able to recognize the inappropriate state, and then be able to change your breath pattern.

At first glance, it would seem obvious that we ought to develop this faculty: to change from the tension state to the relaxed state, and most times this will be the case. However, according to the demands of the situation, the opposite may be appropriate.

There is an optimum state of arousal for every situation.

For instance, you have to make an unpleasant phone call. You really don't want to make it, but it must be done. If you have just had a very pleasant lunch in congenial surroundings and feel very relaxed and at peace with the world, you may very well use breath activation to complete the undesirable task.

The secret of performance in any situation, given that we have the basic tools and training required to meet the challenge, lies in our control over our inner climate. We need to be able to respond appropriately, not just blindly (or react biologically). The first step toward this control is to become consciously aware of our breathing.

We can do without food for long periods and even without water for some time, but we can't sustain life for more than a few minutes without air. Because breath is so essential, so close and intimate, it is the fastest pathway to our inner climate.

The conscious awareness of breathing has to be developed gradually and systematically. For the whole of our life so far we have learned, by default, to ignore rather than to explore it. Before exploring some of the subtle, dynamic potential of breath-to-brain function, let's examine the more basic, but often little understood, mechanics of breathing.

## THE MECHANICS OF BREATHING

Most people think the prime mover in the breathing process is the structure of the chest. You expand your chest and draw in the air, but this is grossly inaccurate. Mechanically speaking, the diaphragm is the initiator. This large sheet of muscle divides the trunk into the thoracic (chest) and abdominal (belly) chambers (see Figure 7A and 7B).

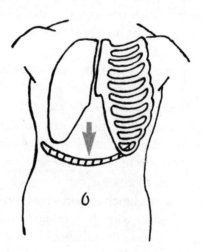

Figure 7A

*Diaphragm during inhalation*

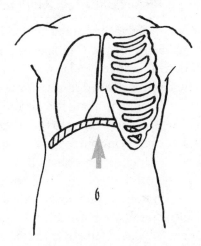

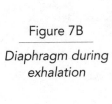

Figure 7B

*Diaphragm during
exhalation*

The diaphragm moves downward, creating positive pressure in the abdominal section and a partial vacuum in the thoracic section. As long as the airway is open, atmospheric pressure forces the air into the lungs. Of course, this process is assisted further, in a muscular sense, by the expanding chest. The action of chest expansion is primarily effected by the intercostal muscles (between the ribs).

When pressure is applied to the abdominal section by the downward movement of the diaphragm, that pressure is relieved by an expansion of the abdominal wall.

If you have ever watched a young baby dozing, you have seen that the baby's chest is hardly involved at all in the breathing process. The only evidence of breathing appears to be the navel rising and falling.

As you inhale, your lungs inflate within the thoracic cavity until they are full, and pressure is equalized with the atmosphere outside. At this point, there is considerable pressure on the heart. That pressure is relieved as you exhale.

The phenomenon of intrathoracic pressure variation is now used in patients recuperating from heart attacks. Patients are taught to control their breathing and to consciously extend the period of exhalation. This makes the work of the heart much easier.

## BRAIN BREATHING: POET OR POLITICIAN

More than just your personal air conditioner, your nose is also your personal brain-function barometer. The flow of your breath through your nostrils is directly related to your brain function.

The brain is divided into two distinct hemispheres with a thin unifying membrane along the middle. To the eye, the hemispheres seem like exact duplicates. In fact, there is some duplication of function, but each hemisphere has its own area of specialization in the processing of sensory information.

The right brain is concerned with spatial perception: imagery, creativity, intuition, and dream-oriented processes. It is not primarily logical, rational, analytical, or sequential in its approach. I call it the Poet. The left brain, in contradistinction, is the Politician. It is rational, analytical, calculating, logical, and sequential in its approach.

At any given moment of the day, either the Poet or the Politician is dominant. This dominance alternates according to a specific rhythm.

It is as if, for example, you were in an auto rally, with driver and co-driver. One is driving, steering, changing gears, braking, and accelerating. The other is taking a rest until it is time to jump into the driver's seat. This is not to say that the co-driver isn't functioning; she may be dozing or noting the changing scenery, but the level of function, although it may be complementary, is not controlling the journey.

At any given moment of this alternating hemispherical dominance, you are more ideally oriented to the performance of tasks by either the Poet or the Politician. How often have you noticed you are drawn irresistibly to doodle with a pencil while the detailed statistical analysis lies off at one side of your desk, silently screaming to be completed?

The dominance alternates, in regular periods of approximately one hour and twenty minutes, throughout the twenty-four hours of your day. The period may vary a little from individual to individual, but the regularity is a well-documented fact. It is biorhythm on a fine and subtle scale, but with potentially great effects in terms of stress.

Due to the structure and organization of our lives in modern times, problems can and do arise from this Poet/Politician alternation. We begin work at a fixed time and we finish at a fixed time (in some cases), and there are certain tasks that must be done within that framework. If the task demands one type of brain function and we are in the other mode, we have stress.

There are times when you have a task to perform—drafting a proposal, doing calculations, making an important phone call—and you just cannot seem to make yourself do it. You look for anything else to do but that! The reason may not be that you are ducking the issue or shirking the task, but rather that your brain is not in the appropriate functional mode.

One wonderful aspect of getting in touch with the body on more subtle levels is that you can tell whether the Poet or the Politician is in charge. Not only can you determine which hemisphere is in control, but you can change it.

## WHO'S IN THE DRIVER'S SEAT?

I have a strong childhood memory of a painting of an Australian aboriginal warrior, standing on one leg. His other leg is raised and bent, with the sole of his foot resting on the knee of the leg supporting his weight. He uses his spear for balance and support. He stands on top of a ridge looking out over a vast plain, and I've often wondered: What is he doing there?

I can't recall which leg he is standing on, but, if I knew, I could tell whether he is immersed in an ancient "Dream Time" vision, or is simply hunting—searching keenly for signs of game. At any given moment, the dominant hemisphere will be reflected in the volume of the breath passing through one or other of the nostrils. If the flow is stronger in the right nostril, the left hemisphere is dominant and, conversely, if the flow is stronger in the left nostril, the right hemisphere is dominant.

You can determine this by moistening a finger and checking from side to side to see which is stronger. With practice and fine-tuning, you can do it mentally.

How often have you had the experience, while suffering from a head cold, of one nostril being totally blocked? After some time you are alerted to the sensation of that nostril clearing, and starting to flow freely, and you think that the cold is almost cured but, alas, within a few seconds, the opposite nostril is totally blocked. All that has happened is a change of drivers up on top!

## How to Change Drivers

By changing the predominant flow in the nostrils, you can directly affect which hemisphere is in control. This can be done purely by blocking the nostril with cotton wool or closing it with the finger or, more subtly, by mentally focusing on the side you wish to accentuate while pressing the tongue firmly against the roof of the mouth on the side you wish to close off!

Pressure under the armpit of the side you wish to close will also augment the process. You can apply this pressure quite unobtrusively by placing your opposite fist in the armpit and consciously squeezing your arm against it.

By transferring your body weight to the nostril side you wish to open and balancing on one leg (like my aboriginal warrior), you can also "change drivers." Interfering with your natural hemisphere rhythm is both possible and permissible, but, particularly in cases where extreme mechanical measures are taken, such as blocking the nostril with cotton wool, the obstruction must be removed while eating and sleeping, so your natural balance can be restored.

I have instructed high school students preparing for exams in these pathways of the breath. They have been able to consciously alter their brain function to the appropriate mode for the particular exam with excellent results, and with greatly reduced stress!

# CHAPTER 8

## The Centering Breath

THIS PRACTICE IS SO essential to the mastery of stress that if you develop and use only this technique, you will have gained a rare and valuable instrument in your toolbox for living.

The Centering Breath can be used any time, in activity or at rest. It is a very intimate and private connection with your vital, dominant brain function, and it is completely unobtrusive; no one else need know that you are doing it.

In the previous chapter, the phenomenon of alternating dominant brain hemispheres was discussed: how the inappropriate situation coupled with the countervailing hemisphere can cause stress, and how it may also be manipulated to reduce that stress. What has yet to be explored is bringing both hemispheres into balanced and equal function, thereby making available, simultaneously, the qualities and special capacities of each. The Centering Breath not only creates the possibility for this to occur, but also immediately initiates changes in your nervous system and blood chemistry, activating the Relaxation Response.

There are separate and distinct components you can quickly learn and then combine to produce the overall effect. The first of these is an ancient, powerful, and subtle form of yoga breathing. Its Sanskrit name is "Ujjayi," but I prefer to call it the Monitoring Breath.

## THE MONITORING BREATH

At the base of your throat there is a small door, or flap (called the epiglottis), which closes when you swallow to prevent food or liquids from entering the trachea, or windpipe. This is a reflex action, an unconscious mechanism, but one you can easily learn to control.

First breathe in, slowly, gently and not too deeply through the nose (keeping the mouth closed) while you are reading this. Become aware of the movement of the air, not in the nostrils, but rather in the throat. Mentally locate this point in the throat where the air enters your windpipe.

When you are ready, while breathing in, slowly and consciously close the epiglottis to prevent the air from going in any farther— just for a second or two. Then open it again, but not fully, and continue your inhalation. When you keep this doorway only partially open, the volume of the air entering the windpipe is reduced and this produces a subtle sound, like an internal rustle or whisper.

Practice keeping the flap steadily in the partially open position (just so you are aware of the sound it produces) while breathing both in and out. Initially, make the sound quite pronounced so that you can easily follow it. You may find it easier to produce the sound on either the inward or the outward breath, but gently work at it until you can establish sufficient control, and make the sound more or less at the same volume, in both phases.

This control is easily mastered if you don't try too hard. Remember that it is a very gentle and subtle technique. If you find yourself short of breath, you are trying too hard. Relax into it. Progressively, you can reduce the sound to a level that is undetectable by anyone else but you.

Even though you are partly externalized reading these instructions, the main focus of your awareness and sensitivity is at the throat, feeling the movement of the air and listening to the sound it makes. The aim of the monitoring phase of the Centering Breath is developing such control that the sound remains perfectly even and smooth during both your inhalation and exhalation. It should also become so relaxed that you feel you could continue with it indefinitely.

As you continue with the monitoring breath you will feel your respiration rate slow down, and you will become more relaxed and calm. You may develop some small discomfort or dryness in the throat. This usually means you are not practicing subtly or gently enough. Don't be too concerned, as the dryness will be eliminated as you develop the next stages of the Centering Breath.

A sign of great success—and this can happen within the first few minutes—is a distinct sensation of coolness at the base of your throat. Sometimes this can be a very pleasant, soothing sensation, what is poetically described as a "silvery sweet radiance."

When you begin to master this aspect of the Centering Breath, the soothing, reflex sensation is transmitted from very sensitive nerve endings in the throat area, called the carotid sinus receptors, to an essential part of the brain. This area is called the reticular activating system, or RAS, and it sits at the top of the spinal cord. This center is responsible for monitoring and adjusting dimensions of your internal climate, such as breathing rate, blood pressure, heart rate, and skin temperature.

The soothing reflex sensation generated by the monitoring breath is transmitted along the nerve pathways to this group of specialized cells. Quite swiftly, it activates the parasympathetic nervous system, or Relaxation Response. It is not uncommon for your breathing rate to drop to around five or six breaths per minute and, with consistent practice, it can go even lower. As you establish the inner climate of relaxation your oxygen consumption will reduce, as your body's ability to take up what fuel it requires increases.

If you suffer from high blood pressure (hypertension), the monitoring breath is the single most significant technique for managing your condition. I have known patients who were virtually confined to bed with severe hypertension, who were able to achieve a full recovery and lead a completely normal life simply by using the Monitoring Breath in combination with Conscious Relaxation.

The second and final stage of the Centering Breath is the means whereby you combine the benefits of the monitoring breath with an even more subtle and intimate process of adjusting brain function by the action of your tongue, called the Tongue Lock.

IN THIS PHASE, EXTEND your tongue gently, inside your closed mouth, so that the tip of your tongue rests against the roof of your mouth.

**MASTERY SOLUTIONS IN PRACTICE:**

**The Tongue Lock**

Explore the roof of your mouth and be aware first of the hard palate, and then the softer part behind it.

During this practice you will keep contact with the roof of the mouth for some time, and your tongue muscles, which are not used to this, can become tired. Whenever you experience any "tongue fatigue," simply rest for a few moments. The contact of the tip of the tongue with the roof of the mouth should be gentle and not involve any great exertion. If you can comfortably reach and hold the tip at the soft palate, that's fine, but your comfort and the capacity to maintain contact is the most important aspect.

To progress to the final stage of the Centering Breath, first complete the monitoring phase effortlessly, so it's almost an unconscious process. Your awareness should remain attached to the internal sound, monitoring the regularity and evenness of the flow of your breath. The rest is a matter of enhancing your internal sensitivity, and you may have to use a degree of imagination at first to achieve a rhythm and mental flow that will produce the proper results.

Slide the tip of your tongue slightly right of the center of the roof of your mouth and exert a gentle pressure there. Bring your awareness to the left nostril and inhale slowly, using the monitoring breath, while feeling that you are breathing exclusively in this nostril only. Focus clearly on the sensation of air moving in your left nostril.

As you reach the top of the inhalation, consciously slide the tip of the tongue over to the left side of the roof of your mouth, and exert a gentle pressure there. As you commence to breathe out, focus exclusively on the outflow of the breath through the right nostril. When you reach the end of the exhalation, keep the tongue pressed gently there, against the left side of the roof of the mouth, and inhale back through the right nostril again.

When you reach the top of the inhalation, slide your tongue over to the right side again and breathe out through your left nostril. This constitutes one complete round of the Centering Breath.

If you wish, you can deepen your experience of this technique by using your imagination. Extending your mental awareness of your breath as it travels along its pathways up into the brain itself. This is a considerably more intense aspect of the technique and relates to the esoteric symbolism of the ancient Egyptian "Ankh." It is an extremely potent Kundalini meditation technique that, by balancing the flow of prana, or bioelectrical energy, in the "everyday" channels, encourages flow in the central channel (Sanskrit term, *Sushumna*). It should be noted that this central channel has to be activated for more energy to be available in awakening dormant areas of the brain.

At this level of practice, you simply continue your mental journey of sensitivity in through the left nostril and up into the right side of your head with each inhalation. As the inhalation reaches its peak and your tongue slides over to the left side of the roof of your mouth, your awareness travels up and over the curved inner surface of your head and into the left side. There it descends, down and out the right nostril—and so on.

Eventually, when you've established balance in the flow of your breath, hold your tongue centrally, and the twin streams of breath will simply follow to and from their subtle merging point, behind the center of your mid-eyebrow.

The Centering Breath brings both hemispheres of the brain into balanced function, making the specialized capacities of each side simultaneously available to you. You can vary the results of the practice according to the situation, as it is also possible to emphasize one side over the other to wake up the more appropriate driver!

The applications of the Centering Breath are almost infinite in terms of effectively managing stress. If you find yourself in a confrontation or an anxiety-producing situation, you can drop into this mode, without concerning yourself with the complexities of the alternating nostril awareness. Merely practice the monitoring breath while keeping your tongue locked right in the middle.

This provides a "breathing space," a pause. In any confrontation where there is aggression or anger, the "fight or flight" mechanism will be instantaneously activated. Your blood chemistry will change suddenly and dramatically, preparing you to either fight back or escape. If the situation involves a superior at work, a valued client, or a customer raging at the complaints desk, it will probably be inappropriate for you to do either. In these situations, what you need to do is respond. This is a conscious and considered act, not just a blind and unconscious reaction. By using the Centering Breath, you create the pause in which you establish chemical and hormonal control. You observe and analyze, planning the best and most appropriate response and, in this way, you cease to be a victim. You become a conscious, rather than a reactive, participant. This gives you a great advantage.

However, unless you have made the tool your own to the degree that it is an automatic mechanism, you will forget to use it. The only way to do this is by practicing it. After the storm has passed, you remember "I should have used the Centering Breath." It does little good to intellectually understand and accept the inherent value of this approach. What makes the method valuable is practice and familiarity.

Remember to use the Six Events described in Chapter 15, "Stress Management Routines" to program this method so deeply that it becomes a natural and unobtrusive way of breathing throughout your day. Use it while driving, traveling on a train, waiting for a bus, between appointments, or before making a presentation.

# CHAPTER 9

# Food for Thought—and Action

WHAT YOU EAT, HOW you eat, when and where you eat will tremendously affect your ability to perform well. If you are expected to perform at a consistently high level throughout the day, and your digestive processes negatively affects that performance, then you will increase your stress.

Let's look at some facts about diet, eating, digestion, and elimination. Food goes in one end, and waste (what we don't either use or store) comes out at the other. During this journey, the body sorts and attends specifically to different food components. If you have a basic understanding of the process, you will be better able to adjust your diet to your individual needs. You can eat to enhance your performance.

The digestive tract can be divided into four sections:

1. The upper section, consisting of your mouth and throat. Digestion begins in your mouth with enzymes secreted in your saliva.

2. The stomach, a living laboratory flask full of acid, which mainly breaks down protein.

3. The small intestine, the longest part of the intestine, which digests carbohydrates.

4. The large intestine, or colon, where the waste is prepared for elimination.

## THE PROTEIN MYTH

Initial research into the minimum daily requirement (MDR) of protein was done in Germany around the turn of the twentieth century. For about sixty years prior to the study, the dietary recommendations were from 125 grams to 175 grams per day. During this period, the Western countries enjoyed increasing affluence. Protein, in the form of meat products (which had always been more expensive than grains, fruit, and vegetables), became much more accessible to the average person. The official promotion and availability of a high proportion of meat in the daily diet prevailed. During this period (except a radical decrease in per capita meat consumption between the two World Wars), there was a dramatic increase in the incidence of heart disease.

Then, in the early 1960s, researchers in Japan, Switzerland, the U.S.A., and around the world tried to replicate the original German research results and were unable to do so. There had been some basic errors in the original procedures. Their subsequent results were between 45 and 80 grams per day, or, in approximate terms, about one third of the original findings.

Excess protein in your diet is one of the major contributors to the increasingly high incidence of coronary heart disease. The byproducts of a protein metabolism, unless discharged (mainly through muscular activity), are toxins. They build up in the muscle tissue, and interfere with its performance. Remember, your heart is a muscle.

Part of the protein myth comes from the erroneous assumptions that, given the human organism's need for a specific spectrum of amino acids (what has been called "complete protein"), this could only be obtained from meat. The reality is that a combination of foods taken at the same meal can provide this range of nutrients, and meat need not be included.

There are pure carnivores, such as cats, dogs, lions, and tigers, and also pure herbivores, like cows and sheep. Humans have some of the characteristics of both groups and are generally classified as omnivores. We will eat anything. A glance at the contents of the table at any seven-year-old's birthday party will immediately confirm this!

Pure carnivores have a high concentration of hydrochloric acid in their stomachs, and they also have a very short intestine. This combination allows them to quickly break down the protein, bone, and sinew, and then excrete the waste very quickly.

Human stomach acid is five times weaker and the intestine is five times longer than that of carnivores. The intestine length is specifically provided for digesting carbohydrates. Mathematically speaking then, it follows logically that if we wish to include meat in our diet, it should proportionately constitute about a fifth (20%) of the intake of carnivores.

There are other factors that contribute to low performance in pure carnivores. For example, what happens immediately after a tiger has a good meal? It goes to sleep for up to twelve hours! The same thing used to happen to our family at my grandfather's house on Christmas day. After a feast of pork, lamb, chicken, etc., (and those were just the hot meats), washed down with copious quantities of different alcoholic beverages, I clearly recall tiptoeing through a very large, darkened house. All the curtains were drawn by 3 P.M., while outside the sun shone through a clear Australian summer afternoon. In every room there were adults, collapsed on beds or slumped in armchairs—the only sound a cacophony of snoring.

If you need to be mentally or physically active, then you simply can't afford to load your digestive system with heavy, high-protein food—particularly at lunch time, because you have to perform for another four to six hours. Compound a high-protein lunch with alcohol, and you deliberately make yourself a candidate for the Twilight Zone. By 3 P.M. you are walking under water. You'll really feel like taking a nap while that important meeting with a valuable client or that detailed analysis you assured your boss would be on her desk by close of business goes by the wayside.

Excess protein contributes to the maintenance of muscular tension. It has a cumulatively damaging effect on your heart. It is a stress factor!

An interesting chemical fact is that the amino acid tyrosine, which forms adrenaline (the stress hormone), is highly concentrated in meat, while tryptophane, which makes serotonin (the relaxation chemical), is plentiful in vegetarian diets.

My purpose here is to provide information and suggestions, not convert you to a totally vegetarian diet. You can, systematically and gradually, make the change to a truly high-performance dietary system. There are some basic rules for eating positively, and we will come to those a little later.

First, let's look more closely at the process of digestion, each step through your body.

Now, assuming that you have chosen a pleasing, well-balanced meal, you bite, chew, and swallow. It used to be said that you should chew each mouthful twenty or thirty times. This assists with the primary digestion, the secretion of salivary enzymes. It may not be the most efficient use of your time. But if you can at least chew the first mouthful until it is a liquid, you will have greatly enhanced the efficiency of the entire digestive process.

Next, the masticated, swallowed food reaches the stomach. The stomach is a bag of living tissue containing acid. It's protected from the corrosive effect of this acid by mucous secreted in its walls. The efficiency of this protective mucous secretion is dependent on the blood supply available to the stomach wall.

Consequently, the blood supply available is dependent on your state of arousal. If your are tense, anxious, afraid, or angry, there is less volume of blood available, less protection, and a higher probability of ulceration (gastric ulcer). Recently, gastric ulcer therapy has been revolutionized by the discovery of a specific causative bacterium. The higher the protein content of the swallowed food, the more acid is required to break it down, and the longer it needs to remain in the stomach.

In the next phase, the partly digested food leaves the stomach and enters the upper part of the small intestine. The mass leaving the stomach is combined with acid and needs to be very quickly neutralized.

Bile, made by the liver and stored in the gall bladder, mixes with the food. The harmful acids are neutralized and the surface tension of the fats is altered (just like detergent in the dishwater). The quality and quantity of the bile and the liver function that provides it are also dependent on optimum blood supply to the area. So if you are tense, anxious, frightened, or angry, there is less blood, less protection, and a higher probability of duodenal ulcer as stomach acids are not effectively neutralized.

As the food continues on its way through the small intestine, messages are sent from sensors in its lining to the pancreas, which secretes insulin. The capacity of the pancreas to function depends on the demands made on it. If you are constantly nibbling away at sweets and eat a lot of processed foods, the pancreas is going to be overworked and will eventually be impaired, especially if you are genetically predisposed to diabetes.

During its journey through the small intestine, the digested food undergoes the process of carbohydrate digestion. By the time the residue reaches the beginning of the large intestine or colon, digestion is virtually complete and, from here on out, the emphasis is on elimination.

Once food has been digested, once you have taken from it what you need, then the imperative becomes to get rid of the waste as quickly and easily as possible. However, there is still some valuable material left in the mass, such as water, salts, etc., in solution. So this next phase is the removal through the colon wall of what your body can recycle. The question of elimination is so important and the function of the colon so essential that the following figures are worth considering.

In the first part, the ascending colon, waste has to travel uphill, against gravity. It reaches a corner, called the hepatic flexure (because it is near the liver), then travels down and across the transverse colon and up to another corner, called the splenic flexure (near the spleen). From there it is all downhill to the point of expulsion.

Whenever you see a person with a "beer belly," their colon probably looks like that in Figure 9A. A diet of junk food, frequent overeating, and a largely sedentary lifestyle cause the muscular wall of the abdomen to protrude and sag. The transverse colon also sags down, partially closing off the two corners or flexures.

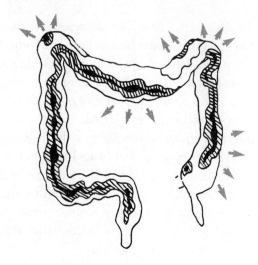

Figure 9A

*An Unhealthy
Colon*

This results in a buildup of, you will remember, toxic material, just before both flexures, and also in the lower part of the transverse colon. If you recall that the function of this whole pipe is absorption, then it's easy to see how there may be leakage of this toxic material indicated by the arrows in Figure 9A.

Constipation can be both a result and a cause in this situation, a process of self-poisoning. Unwanted chemicals, preservatives, etc. and the toxic byproducts of metabolism are absorbed back into the system. These byproducts affect the liver, spleen, pancreas, uterus and ovaries, prostate, and the brain.

Constipation almost deserves a chapter to itself, but let's keep to these few observations. This condition can be a cause and a result of stress. We are civilized and sophisticated beings, and progressively less in touch with our basic bodily processes.

About twenty minutes after consuming a substantial meal, we experience an urge to eliminate (called the gastro-colic reflex). Trouble begins when we override this message for convenience. The message is repeated at a few intervals, but each time it is ignored, it gets weaker, until it finally stops.

"Normal bowel frequency" is based on general observation, not on what happens in a healthy, happy person. So, you are not considered to be constipated if you have one daily bowel movement, or even if

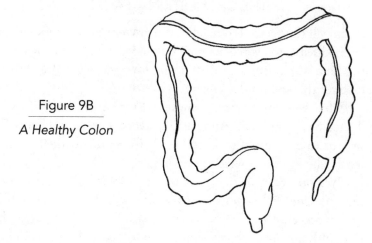

Figure 9B

*A Healthy Colon*

you have one every second day. The truth is that the ideal frequency is in direct and natural relation to the number of meals you eat.

Of course, food quality is very important in maintaining regularity, but mental and emotional factors can be even more so. Constipation can prevail, even with frequent and regular exercise and a good quality high-fiber diet. It is directly related to your inner tension and to stress left unmanaged.

Headaches are a classic byproduct of constipation. The toxins circulating in the bloodstream directly affect brain function. Also, strong body odor, bad breath, and skin irritation are also common. This is simply because the other eliminative organs, your skin and lungs, have to take up the job of eliminating toxins.

All of these symptoms of constipation can be significant stress factors in themselves, adding to the problem, and maintaining a cycle that must be interrupted for you to be fully vital and achieve your highest levels of performance.

How can you interrupt this cycle? Learn to relax. Get in touch with the complex and wonderful vehicle that carries your mind around, and become aware of the messages your vehicle sends to you, the driver. Eat food you enjoy and create a state of enjoyment while eating.

## THE CHOLESTEROL FACTOR

Although this factor is crucial in the prevention of heart and circulatory disease, we won't examine it in any detail, because research in this area is an ongoing process. I will, however, leave you with some food for thought on the subject.

A few years ago a very comprehensive survey was jointly conducted by Scottish and Australian university medical schools. They set out to examine the effects of totally removing dietary cholesterol. Their findings were astounding.

Over one year, research volunteers avoided all dietary cholesterol. Progressively, over the first several months of the experiment, their blood cholesterol dropped dramatically. Later in the year, however, although the subjects continued to avoid all forms of cholesterol, their levels began to inexorably climb again until at the end of the study, they were virtually the same as when they had begun.

While we should obviously use care and moderation in this one aspect of our diet, it is the cholesterol we produce internally that can constitute the real problem. If we understand that cholesterol production is significantly altered by stress and take appropriate measures to reduce the effect of stress, we are positively addressing the cholesterol question also.

## SOME SIMPLE RULES

1. Exercise your legs (stair-climbing is excellent) before eating, then sit quietly for a few minutes before beginning to eat. Sit quietly for a minimum of five minutes after eating.

2. When you eat, just eat. Don't talk or read. You can afford at least fifteen minutes for this.

3. Chew the first mouthful until it is liquid. Get in touch. Don't eat mindlessly.

4. Never eat when you are angry or anxious.

5. Be consistent in your eating habits.

6. Take charge of your lunch hour. It is the most important period of your day in terms of maintaining a high performance level.

7. Determine your blood type and read Dr. Peter J. D'Adamo's *Eat Right For Your Type*, a helpful guide to food groups.

## THE HIGH PERFORMANCE LUNCH HOUR

It is probably more appropriate to call this period lunch "time" rather than lunch "hour," as it's not uncommon these days to have considerably less than an hour of personal time available in the middle of the day. Sometimes your lunch hour may be only twenty minutes. Even so, planning how you spend this time, whatever its duration, can have a significant effect on your performance for the remainder of the day.

It doesn't matter whether you are a sales representative driving from one appointment to the next, working in a crowded "open plan" office situation, on a factory floor, a parent at home with young children, or a manager with your own personal office, the potential for lunch time to make or break your afternoon needs to be understood.

We have just examined in some detail what you should eat and what you should avoid, particularly at lunch time. It is a simple biological fact that a heavy, high-protein lunch makes you drowsy and can severely impair your performance. A greater volume of blood is drawn to your stomach, and less is available to the brain. This will affect your levels of attention and concentration.

If you compound a meal of this sort by drinking alcohol, chances are you will not be of great value to yourself, your company or family and, by mid-afternoon when your biological processes are naturally at a lower level, you may be a liability.

### Climate Control Before the Meal

If your morning has been stressful, if there has been pressure, confrontation, or anxiety, then you need to resolve your internal chemical climate before you take any food at all. If this is your condition at lunch time, then internally a greater volume of blood will be drawn away from the stomach, leaving it less protected against its own acidic secretions. Eating when you are tense is creating the perfect situation for gastric ulcers.

You can change the inner climate very quickly by using techniques such as the Humming Bee, Letting Go, and the Centering Breath (see more in Practices 3, 5, and Chapter 8). Use whatever combination suits your time and situation.

If you can chew your first mouthful until it is completely liquid, you will efficiently prime your digestive system to perform at its optimum.

Rather than dwelling on the "lunch" aspect of the break, it's worthwhile to examine it as planned stress management, and to focus on getting the most value from your time in terms of your overall well-being and your subsequent performance.

### Getting Away Somewhere

This doesn't mean you should run through the city like a headless chicken, paying accounts, doing shopping, and generally exhausting yourself by the time you have to return to your job. If you have only twenty minutes, take five of them to walk outside your building, to breathe deeply and look around, particularly up at the sky. Even if you are in the middle of an industrial park or a huge factory complex, the sky will bring you relief and exercise your faculty of sight while it soothes the mind—even if the sky is gray and overcast. If you can't leave the building, go exploring through other floors, using stairs whenever possible.

If a park is nearby, go there and take your shoes off for a few minutes and walk barefoot on the grass. This is not only a pleasurable and relaxing activity, it is bioelectrically therapeutic. All modern manmade structures create electromagnetic fields that have a subtle but powerful and cumulative effect on those who are confined for long periods within them. If computers are a significant factor in your workplace, then this condition is compounded. Walking bare-foot for even a few minutes restores the body's natural electromag-netic balance. It literally grounds you, electrically.

Of course, if it is snowing outside, you will have to adapt your program accordingly. Make contact with trees (even if their branches are bare), or handle any living plants available to you. The change from an insulated, ionically positive environment to expo-sure to the natural elements, for even a few minutes, regardless of the weather, is always worthwhile.

## Drop In and Say Hello

Although it may be socially stimulating, or even relaxing, to spend some time with your fellow workers, the person you most need to make contact with, and who will benefit most from that contact—is you!

If you have been externalized all morning and meeting chal-lenges, you will derive tremendous benefit from even a few minutes of withdrawal from external experience and spending some time with yourself, to the exclusion of all other activity. Use the Relax-ation Pose (see Practice 9) if the situation permits, or the Centering Breath (see more information in Chapter 8).

The beauty of entering the borderline state generated by these techniques is that an internal chemical climate is quickly estab-lished that discharges accumulated muscular tension, and allows your body—and your mind—to restore and repair itself on a cellular level. The result is greater mental and physical energy, available for your afternoon. Lunchtime then becomes a mini-holiday from which you emerge refreshed and better prepared to deal with the rest of your day.

Lunchtime is not a time to continue working without a break. If you are serious, both about performing at optimum and maximizing your potential for health and enjoyment, then this is using time well, and is crucial to these goals. Plan your lunch break as seriously as you would plan any other aspect of your working life.

## CHAPTER 10

# Ethics, Personal and Professional

AN ATTENTION TO ETHICS in business, and indeed in life, is essential to the effective management of stress. It is worthwhile for you to give some consideration to this question, and to express your conclusions by clearly formulating your code, whether as a corporate entity, or as an individual.

It is not important if your code is based on religious morality, an intuitive understanding of the essential interdependence of all living beings, or simply on the practicality of being ethical in all your dealings. What is important is that you are clear about, comfortable with, and committed to your code as a standard by which to live and work.

## ETHICS IS A HEALTH ISSUE

*The sum of the ethics of the individuals who comprise a business will be, sooner or later, for better or worse, the ethics of that organization.*
—Geoffrey Garrott
from *Ethics in Business: A Deeper Approach*

Our community, be it business or social, is as healthy as it is ethical. The degree to which ethics are practiced, in personal or business life, is a major determinant of underlying stress levels.

In business, applied ethical standards provide a reasonable expectation of behavior that can be relied upon in any transaction. If there are no such standards, all dealings become vague, and consequently, complex and stressful.

When I say all commerce, I refer not solely to the interaction between businesses and professions, but to the whole structure of corporate function. From the CEO, through the entire framework of management and staff, to the client or consumer, these standards can, if practiced, bring health and vitality to the business and to each of its human components—even your competitors!

We may have been trained and educated to be accountants, managers, truck drivers, and tennis players, but we may not have been trained and educated to be fulfilled and functional human beings. Educating people for the most essential aspect of life, that of *relationship,* is still in its infancy, because society's focus has been inefficiently utilitarian.

I say "inefficiently" because, no matter how pragmatically comprehensive our training and education has been, the very foundation is inadequate. If we are in any way impaired, and we are, then the whole society is also dysfunctional to a degree that is compounded by, and not merely the sum total, of that dysfunction. The whole question of relationship, both interpersonal and especially in the world of commerce, is still largely unaddressed. The ramifications of impaired relationships spread like ripples of disease throughout society.

Healthy relationships have, at their core, the basic principle of applied ethics, the principle of service.

## The Principle of Service

When it is consistently applied to all dimensions of relationship, service is a liberating, empowering and life-promoting force, not some dry philosophical or moral theory.

Interaction with colleagues, superiors, clients, consumers, shopkeepers, and bus drivers, not to mention friends and family, can be sustained, nurtured and turned into an ongoing process of life-affirmation. It can be a source of endless satisfaction and joy, if you can embrace the idea and make it a reality.

Whether you intend to climb the corporate ladder or do the dishes, make decisions that may affect a workforce of hundreds or choose new school uniforms for children, the awakening of a deep and vitalizing sense of purpose and awareness can be brought about by approaching all your relationships from the practice of service.

## The Practice of Service

To live your life from the platform of service involves two processes. The first is to stop and honestly look at yourself: what you want from life, your expectations of others, what makes you feel loved, happy and secure and, most importantly, what you are prepared to do or give in order to actualize your desires, passions, and ambitions.

This analysis is essential if you want to be a fulfilled human being. If you haven't taken stock in this way, then formulated your approach to the rest of your life (always an unknown quantum), it is highly likely that you will continue to blunder through it, driven by unconscious action and blind conditioning.

This first step in actualizing the principle of service is being conscious of your situation. It is a complex and comprehensive analysis, not completed over a cup of coffee, but one that may take some days or weeks. As your aims and needs begin to crystallize, you will see how deeply these forces in your life depend on and affect others!

Unless you have an exclusively egocentric perception of life (in which case you would be so stressed by dissatisfaction and frustration that it's unlikely you would even bother to read this chapter), it becomes obvious to you how deeply and unavoidably you are connected to the rest of us: your family, friends, colleagues and ultimately, albeit with diminishing impact as the ripples spread, the whole of humanity.

You are not alone. And, just as you have your needs, ambitions and desires, so does each of us. If you looked at this situation rationally

and were trying to determine the best-case scenario for each of us to
have all our priorities met, you would have to conclude that a prevailing attitude of inflexible selfishness would be the least likely to
promote mutual satisfaction.

## Best and Present Practice

The second step in actualizing the principle of service consists of
two interrelated principles. First, in any situation, whether work,
domestic, or social, you make a conscious commitment to do your
very best, to strive for excellence in all your activities.

The best practice, both in corporate and individual terms, is not
just about the most efficient way of achieving a healthy "bottom
line" (either an acceptable profit, or realized personal goals), it is
about every dimension of activity and how our performance of that
activity affects our business, colleagues, family, friends and society.
It is about giving.

Our individual, and by extension societal, focus seems to have
been rather the opposite of this. We are concerned about getting.
Employees may be focused on what they can get from the company
with the least contribution on their part, and companies may be
similarly and callously oriented. This creates two egocentric and
selfish worlds in collision, pervading all levels of our interaction. As
a direct result, growth, health, and harmony, both in business and
personal spheres, are hamstrung.

Giving (or service) is actually the very root of getting. This
means that an attitude of giving your personal best in all circumstances will inevitably provide a return that can never be matched
by the opposite approach. You continue to grow, and because of the
intense personal satisfaction that follows this mode of conduct, you
will positively glow—whatever may be the short term or immediate
response to your service.

So, it shouldn't matter that those around you may be hell-bent on
squeezing to their personal advantage whatever they can from a situation. Their greed or selfishness is based on ignorance, fear, and insecurity, and is only a symptom of immaturity, whether they are a

corporation or a human being. You cannot and really ought not try to change anyone's perception unless your advice is openly sought.

It is a reality that if you cease to contribute to insecurity, fear and greed and instead direct your investment into positivity and service, then a double effect is produced, however subtly, on the whole human psyche.

In very practical terms, an essential component of service is that you be here! When you consciously lift yourself and remain fully present and aware in the moment, you are truly alive. Much of our life is spent, and in many cases actually wasted, by mentally being somewhere else or, more usually, some*when* else. You cannot change the past and, in reality, your future is not only unavailable, but is entirely dependent on the present. Life is a series of present moments and, if we miss them or make ourselves unavailable to them by dwelling in fantasy, regret, expectation, or projection, then that is so much life we have not truly lived.

By spending our time at work and wishing we were somewhere else, looking forward to payday, or the weekend, or the annual holidays, we make it impossible to perform at our best and, in the process, we actually cheat ourselves of the true experience of real life as it unfolds moment to moment.

This process of gaining awareness or sharpening your consciousness where you are totally present is not accomplished overnight. We must transcend a tremendous inertia. This inertia is the sum of the conditioned thought patterns and attention developed over a lifetime.

There are tools you can used to guide your awareness. The practices of Inner Silence and Body Check (see Chapter 5) and the Centering Breath (see Chapter 8) are a few. By using the Six Events (see Chapter 15, "Stress Management Routines") you can make the process of "waking up" (or "coming alive") a gradual and progressively rewarding experience. As you practice and enjoy the state of increasing wakefulness, the old patterns will drop away by themselves.

Often, when we are striving for excellence in any activity, there is an implicit expectation of a particular result. When events or circumstances prevent the expected result from occurring, we feel disappointment and frustration, and ultimately, stress. However, when you engage in "Best and Present Practice," your focus narrows to the activity at hand and there is always, at the end of the process, the satisfaction that you have done your best, whatever the result.

# CHAPTER 11

# A Mastery of Time

THE ORTHODOXY OF MANAGEMENT training has always been efficiency in performance. It has been the motivation for effective time management. The end result has not changed, but the pathway to its achievement is now illuminated by greater understanding.

The short-term criteria, implicit in the "time and motion analysis," are being replaced with a more comprehensive and long-term view. For example, from a cost-efficient point of view, it can be more sustainable if it is approached on a "user-friendly" basis rather than simply planning it along its most spartan, coldly utilitarian path. If the team is not only intact at completion of a task, but feeling nurtured and valued, the next task—and there is always a 'next'—will be approached with vigor and confidence. In other words, although the distance between two points may not be the shortest if it isn't perfectly straight, it may be more enjoyable and therefore more productive.

Sustainability is the most essential criterion that can be applied to any worthwhile process, whether it be in work practice or your personal life. It's no good to consistently achieve goals in the shortest possible time if, after an indeterminate period (could be six months or five years) you are burnt out, or on sick leave from stress-related illness, and of no use to your company, your family, or yourself.

## PLANNING AND PRIORITIZING

Just as long-range planning for viability and sustainability is now recognized as crucial in any industry, so it is with you. To survive and even succeed, you have to explore and then examine all dimensions of your life in terms of your priorities. You are both the "prime mover" and the ultimate judge in this examination. The specific functional demands of each aspect of your life (work and personal) need to be constantly (that is, daily) reviewed, and your priorities adjusted.

In the old management training approach, it used to be considered sufficient to plan and prioritize (in the workplace only) on a weekly or monthly basis. It set the structure, gave order, and created a blueprint for performance, and thereby a degree of comfort. Now the situation is much more challenging and complex. We understand that we must have, simultaneously, an extremely long-range view that definitely includes our processes of personal relationship, and a daily system of review allowing us to adapt effectively to constantly changing demands.

The choice is yours when establishing the discipline of planning and prioritizing. You may keep an electronic diary, make lists, scribble notes on the palm of your hand, or tie pieces of string around your fingers, but whatever reference system you prefer, the crucial practice is to program a specific time or regular series of moments when you consult your system. If you are a manager with a personal assistant, you can use this resource very efficiently.

Keeping "spontaneously" in touch with home base, contacting your partner at odd and unexpected times ought to be included. Lack of planning of your work activities causes inordinate stress as events and demands pile up haphazardly. Integration of your personal life and relationships in time management is essential to overall planning. If this dimension of your life is not addressed as comprehensively as you plan your work, similar stress is bound to accumulate and this, in turn, will affect your ability to function at work.

## A PLAN FOR TIME MANAGEMENT

In the understanding that stress impairs efficiency, it becomes increasingly important to factor regular periods of stress management into your approach to time management.

### Dealing with Deadlines

The deadline is the embodiment of stress. It ruthlessly determines how much time we have to accomplish a given task and, in providing such an emphatic parameter, can spur us on to achieve magnificently. Conversely, it can be the sword of Damocles hanging over our heads. Deadlines simply must be met, but whether they are well met can only be determined by looking at many different factors.

In all business, but particularly in such industries as finance, advertising, accounting, architecture, journalism and law, the rule is that as soon as one deadline is met, another takes its place. If the individual or the team's resources are depleted after meeting a particularly demanding deadline, they are vulnerable to subsequent lowered performance in meeting the next challenge. Whether the project is a new financial product launch, an advertising campaign, or a submission to the Supreme Court, stress management planning needs to be incorporated into the project's finite timeframe.

When the basketball coach calls timeout with fifteen seconds on the clock and the home team is trailing by two points, this break in the flow of the game can produce startling results. Productive breaks when you're dealing with deadlines can do the same thing.

Remember to plan for regular small periods of relaxation, physical exercise, and occasional longer periods of deep relaxation, especially when the deadline demands an all-night session or a series of late nights. Your health and vitality and that of the team at the end of the process is essential to meet the next challenge.

The powerful stimulus of the deadline and its capacity to bring out the creative best in a team is well understood by anyone who has participated in the process. However, techniques such as deep relaxation and creative visualization are only beginning to be understood in tapping into that well spring of creativity in a more productive and less stressful way. (See Chapter 14, "The Power of

Affirmations" for more information on creative visualization.) Your capacity to concentrate, create and, importantly, to endure is enhanced by planned stress and time management.

## CHAPTER 12

# Bringing It All Back Home

HOW MANY TIMES HAVE you felt or heard your coworkers describe the inability to leave the office *at the office?*

Work and home are two distinct and separate worlds. They need to be distinct and separate, but the reality is that, in most cases, they are worlds in collision! There exists a cycle that can indeed be described as "vicious" where the unmanaged stress at work negatively affects the home environment. The domestic stress caused and perpetuated by this impact, in its turn, has a cumulatively negative effect on work performance, adding to the stress in the office. In the case where you work from a home office and cannot leave the battlefield at the end of the day, this collision can be almost continuous and can lead to dangerous levels of stress. Even if your personal stress management aim is to enhance your job performance and be more successful at your work, you will still need to understand how it interacts with your domestic environment, too.

Although the two worlds are distinct and separate, they are inevitably interconnected. For performance and success on the one hand, and enjoyment, rest, relaxation and a fulfilling personal life on the other, this connection must be accepted. Then appropriate methods of maximizing the opportunities and challenges presented by each can be incorporated into your lifestyle. The first and most practical step is to create an emphatic demarcation point between the two. This is called the "Airlock."

## THE AIRLOCK

People working in potentially highly toxic situations, such as biological laboratories or radioactive environments, are to use a systematic and comprehensive decontamination regimen for industrial safety purposes. The residue of the workplace can also be highly toxic in a mental and emotional as well as physical sense, and if it is brought into your home, it will contaminate your personal life.

If you are single, with no family responsibilities and fewer demands on your personal time, you are in a position to utilize this practice in a very dynamic and life-enhancing way. The earlier in your working life you incorporate such an essential regimen, the easier it will be to maintain it if your domestic situation changes.

In a family situation without a decontamination routine, two waves of stress, each with differing sources, meet each other at the front door and the immediate result is turbulence—confusing what could be a mutually healing and supportive interaction.

Many people, striving unconsciously to create a distinction between home and work, already incorporate a routine that attempts to separate the two sources. The construction workers will adjourn to a bar after a day of pouring concrete and dealing with the demands of a driving and aggressive foreman. Junior executives and managers may adjourn to their preferred bars. The high performer salesperson will enjoy a round of circuit training at the gym, or drop in at the squash court for a workout

But are these attempts to decontaminate the most effective ways to achieve the goal? In most cases they are not, although each may have some merit. One inevitable reality is that the higher you ascend the corporate ladder, the more blurred the distinction between home and work will become. The demands of senior management positions expect that you arrive early and leave late (often taking work home with you) and there is also the tacit expectation that your partner or spouse will also involve him or herself in corporate social functions. Although this tends to apply to more archaic corporate attitudes, the company may view your spouse as an asset or a liability, and it is crucial that you don't hold this perception as there is an implication of prerequisite utility which can denigrate your relationship. Negotiate with your partner for a level of interaction that is supportive of your career path but that doesn't impose any onerous burden.

I know one general manager who discussed the issue of spousal involvement with his wife, an articulate and independent woman with a rich personal life and satisfying career of her own. They compromised and resolved that she would happily attend only three major corporate social functions per year, ones she would be most likely to enjoy, and those of the most significance to his career.

### Creating an Effective Airlock

Discuss with your partner and family your need for a regimen, explaining how it can allow you all to interact positively. When you all understand that life can be much more enjoyable with this regimen, it is easier to establish and maintain the routine.

When you arrive at home, the first step in your decontamination sequence is both symbolic and practical: take a shower. Make it brief and if climate permits, finish with a quick burst of cold water. Follow this with Neti (see Practice 7, page 165), remembering to drain your nostrils effectively.

Go directly to a room or space where you will not be disturbed for twenty minutes, and begin with "Letting Go." This is a superbly efficient technique for releasing both muscular and mental tensions. When you become accomplished at "Letting Go," the practice can be completed in only six minutes.

THE TECHNIQUE CONSISTS OF two aspects: contraction and relaxation. The contraction of each muscle group is made gradually and progressively. Coordinate the action with a slow, deep inhalation through your nostrils,

**MASTERY SOLUTIONS IN PRACTICE:**

**Letting Go**

using a subtle form of the Monitoring Breath. It takes as long to tighten the muscle group as it does to breathe in.

When you reach the top of the inhalation, hold your breath for a count of three while the contraction is maintained at maximum level.

Release your breath, and the accompanying relaxation of the area is totally different from the inhalation and contraction. It is swift and sudden, a matter of instantaneously relinquishing your conscious contraction while allowing your breath to explode through your mouth, with the sound "Pah!"

Your aim is to keep the rest of your body, apart from the area being operated, relaxed and uninvolved with the process. While you are practicing, check from time to time to make sure that you aren't tightening the muscles of your face or tensing your arms too. It takes a little while to acquire the knack.

Here is the practice in sequence: Lie comfortably on your back on the floor, your feet slightly apart and palms upward. Close your eyes. First become aware of your natural breathing and wait a few moments for it to settle down. When it has slowed of its own accord, take in a Monitoring Breath, but very subtly and with hardly any contraction at your epiglottis—just enough to establish control and evenness.

### Right leg

Slowly inhale while tensing all the muscles of the right leg, from the foot to the hip. Begin the contraction by separating the toes and bending the foot back a little, then send it up through the calf, shin, knee and thigh. As the contraction spreads up the leg, raise your leg slightly so that at the top of the breath, the whole stiffened leg is held a few inches above the floor—just enough to give clearance under the thigh muscles.

Hold your breath and contract for the count of three.

Let your breath escape suddenly through your mouth with the explosive sound "Pah" and, simultaneously, let your leg drop to the floor. It is important not to put your leg down, but to suddenly allow it to drop. This means you should also be careful not to raise it too high to avoid hurting your heel.

Begin the process again and repeat a total of three times. Do the same for your left leg.

### Pelvis

As you inhale, progressively tense the muscles of your buttocks and the entire pelvic floor, tightening the anal and urinary sphincter muscles also. Hold the contraction and the breath at maximum for the count of three, then suddenly release the breath, with its accompanying sound, while instantly letting go of the contraction. Repeat three times.

Remember to check your facial muscles and other muscles to ensure that the rest of the body remains uninvolved.

### Belly

As you inhale, feel the air entering deeply into your abdomen, feeling it fill the area. Then, consciously expand your belly like a huge balloon, pushing your navel up towards the ceiling. Hold for the count of three, then release suddenly with the same sound. Repeat three times.

### Chest

Leaving your belly uninvolved, fill and expand the chest as you inhale. This expansion is not just a frontal and upward movement but also a lateral expansion, a spread that you feel at the shoulder blades in the back, and a tightening of the pectoral (breast) muscles. Hold the contraction and the breath for the count of three, then suddenly release with the sound. Repeat three times.

### Right Arm

With your palm upward, inhale slowly and gradually, make a fist of the right hand then send the tightening up through the forearm, elbow, and upper arm. When you reach the top of the breath, the whole stiffened arm is raised and held a few inches above the floor.

Hold your breath for the count of three then suddenly release with the sound, letting your arm drop to the floor and allowing the fist to unclench. Repeat three times. Do the same for your left arm.

## Shoulders

While you inhale and allow your arms to lie slack and uninvolved in the process, raise both shoulders from the floor and try to make them meet in front of your chest. Unless you are unbelievably flexible, it is unlikely that they will. Don't strain in the process. Hold, with the breath, for the count of three, then suddenly release with the sound, letting your shoulders drop back to the floor. Repeat three times.

## Throat and Neck

As you move up to your head, the contractions become progressively more subtle and specific and you reduce the volume of the sound. While inhaling, tense the muscles of the throat and neck. Hold for the count of three then suddenly release with the breath. Repeat three times. The sound "Pah" gradually becomes softer as you move up your head.

## Jaw, Lips, and Cheeks

Inhale and press your lips together more firmly while tensing your cheeks and clenching your jaw. At the top of the breath, hold for the count of three then suddenly release with the sound. Your mouth should drop fully open. Repeat three times.

## Nostrils

While inhaling, consciously tense the nose tip and flare the nostrils. You may also be aware of a sensation at the ears as you do this. Hold for three then suddenly release with the subtle sound. Repeat three times.

## Eyes

There are two aspects of the technique in this area. First, as you inhale, slowly press the upper eyelids down against the lower. Throughout your waking day the muscles that operate the eyelids have been concerned with keeping them open, with occasional relief as you blink. Here you are consciously lowering them and pressing them down in the opposite direction.

Only at the very end of this movement, and at the top of the breath, does the second phase take place. At the top of the breath, while you hold and count to three, all the muscles surrounding your eye sockets are tightened, so that the eyeballs themselves are squeezed. After holding for three, while doing your best to ensure that the rest of the face is not also being contorted, suddenly release with the sound. Repeat three times.

### Forehead and Scalp

As you inhale, keep your eyes closed, raise your eyebrows up towards the hairline, creasing the muscles of the forehead. Also tense the muscles of the whole scalp.

Hold for three counts and release. Repeat three times.

### Whole Body

Slowly inhale and, starting at the toes, gradually apply the contraction upward throughout your entire body. Your legs and arms should be slightly raised. Hold for three counts, then release with the sound. Repeat three times.

This completes the Letting Go sequence. Explore your whole body and try to detect any areas where you are holding residual tension. If you discover any, repeat the appropriate sequence for these areas.

Having discharged the tension throughout the body, spend a few moments just being aware of your natural, uncontrolled breathing.

On completion of the sequence, stand up slowly and practice Shaking All Over (see Practice 1, page 129) for about sixty seconds. Proceed, slowly increasing your pace, into three full rounds of Sun Salutation (see Practice 11, page 193). Lie in the Relaxation Pose (see Practice 9, page 177) for a minute or two until your breathing and heart rate are normal, then sit comfortably and practice a round or two of Brain Massage (see Practice 3, page 143). Focus your thoughts toward family interaction, and then leave the airlock.

The complete sequence can be accomplished in twenty minutes. This small time investment can provide a valuable return.

## THE GIFT OF FRIENDSHIP

In order to live a productive, healthy life unimpaired by stress, it is important that our personal relationships be as stress-free as possible, and that they provide companionship and support. Unless your spouse is a saint (or a self-effacing masochist), this is not going to be the case without some real and conscious effort on your part.

All of the qualities and benefits you would expect to derive from a relationship—feelings of being needed, accepted, loved and supported, opportunities to share triumphs and challenges, to help and be helped—are also required by your partner!

If you are fortunate enough (or have worked at it diligently enough) to be in a caring, warm relationship, it is probable that you already have a high degree of mutual provision in these areas. However, the gift of friendship is not a fixed and finite fact. It is, rather, an ongoing two-way process that must be nurtured and sustained.

The higher the degree of challenge in your life, whether on the home front or in the workplace, the greater the need to attend to this aspect of nurturing. The bases of this nurturing can be summed up as: contact, communication, and attention.

A simple, gentle, and reassuring touch can often defuse a potentially explosive and damaging situation. A ten-second telephone call at an odd time of the day, especially when it is unexpected, to say "thinking of you" or "I love you" can work wonders for you both. Your partner feels "stroked." At the same time, you have re-established your connection with the security of your home base even in the midst of high-pressure work.

"Planned" spontaneity shows that you care. Gifts don't have to be expensive, just thoughtful!

Without communication, a relationship will not survive. In order to communicate, you have to be able to make and sustain contact. You have to be there, physically and mentally. Your body posture and body language should align with your intent. You have to be attentive. Allow yourself to smile, keep eye contact in a relaxed way, and invest your voice with appropriate warmth. Listen to your partner.

It is certain that communication suffers when you're parked in front of the TV, so plan your time at home to reduce what is non-essential, and to augment what is crucial. Turn off the television and meet your partner!

## SEX AND STRESS MANAGEMENT

A fulfilling and mutually nurturing sexual relationship has vast potential for stress management, but only if stress management or stress "relief" is not the prime motivation for sex.

As human beings we are on the highest rung of the evolutionary ladder and sex is no longer simply an opportunity for reproduction, regardless of what fundamentalists of various sorts would have us believe.

Sexual orgasm, and indeed the whole process of sexual arousal and interplay, can produce a significantly altered mental state and biochemistry. Our approach to it is defined and determined by our personality and needs.

At its best it provides an inexhaustible wellspring of energy, insight, and joy. Read Dr. Jonn Mumford's *Ecstasy Through Tantra* (St. Paul: Llewellyn Publications, 1987), for more information. On the mundane, uninspired, and less conscious levels of experience, it brings a brief respite from repetitive, obsessive thought patterns and hormonal thralldom. At its worst, it is the currency of domination, oppression, power, and egocentric abuse.

Although it is neither my purpose here to delve deeply and explicitly into this dimension, nor to provide a manual for sexual expression, I feel that the potential of sex for enhancement of peace, creativity, and the purposeful and conscious enjoyment of our lives remains largely unexplored.

I do understand that, unless approached with courage and consciousness, sexual interaction can be a minefield of negativity that can severely affect your well-being. It may be one of the most significant stress factors in your life! Feelings of being frustrated, unloved, or those of being used or taken for granted can, because the sexual act is so intimately linked with the primitive brain (the limbic system), produce an internal climate of stress that can be very dangerous.

Although it is by no means the most important aspect of a nurturing, mutually supportive relationship, it is, however, a crucial one. Rarely does it happen that sex, like any other dimension of relationship, is spontaneously perfect. Optimum expression and mutual benefit are things you have to work at, by honesty, integrity, consideration, and practice.

The best advice I can give is to accept and remain friends with yourself; be as alert and conscious—present—as you are able and, most of all, remember, as I heard from a psychologist friend many years ago, "At the end of every sexual organ, there dangles a human being."

# CHAPTER 13

## To Sleep, Perchance to Dream

DEEP, RESTORATIVE SLEEP IS important in the day-to-day management of stress. It is crucial to the maintenance of health and vitality, crucial to the maintenance of high levels of productivity and performance, and crucial to survival and sanity.

There are different phases of sleep through which we all pass during the period from eyes closed to eyes open. There are three that need to be understood and positively exploited for effective mastery of stress:

1. The Borderline State
2. The Dream State
3. Deep, Dreamless Sleep

### THE BORDERLINE STATE

We enter the borderline state, also called the hypnogogic state, as we drift off to sleep. The term "drifting" is particularly appropriate to describe this phase, as we are neither awake nor fully asleep. Much of the information brought to the brain through the senses is no longer being consciously registered, and sensations such as weightlessness are quite common.

It is not unusual to experience involuntary, spontaneous muscle movement. Sometimes your arm or leg will twitch or move quite dramatically; sometimes your whole body convulses as if it had risen above the bed and then suddenly dropped back onto the mattress. All of this muscular activity is very normal and usually proportionately related to your degree of stress.

As you relax in this borderline phase, your body's internal chemical and nervous climate also begins to change. Muscle groups, especially in the areas of thighs, arms and abdomen, begin to release their accumulated tension as the nervous and chemical signals that initiated the tension are altered. My personal feeling is that the big "jumps and bumps" are felt because there is a conditioned or habitually maintained defensive state (tension), and the body briefly and spontaneously reverts to that when the physical passivity (which it reads as vulnerability) of relaxation begins to supervene.

Really, all that is happening is that muscular tension, as part of the "Fight or Flight" mechanism, is resolving itself, so you can be assured that it is a healthy indicator.

In fact, one of the two important characteristics of the borderline state is its release of muscular tension, and the subsequent benefits of that muscular relaxation. Establishing and maintaining the borderline state for any length of time, as in the practice of Conscious Relaxation (see Practice 9, page 179, and Chapter 5, "An Antidote for Stress"), can comprehensively resolve your muscular tension.

The second important aspect of the borderline state is the opportunity that it presents for positive autosuggestion. During the state, deeper levels of mind are particularly receptive to information or directives from the conscious mind. (The borderline state is now being utilized in language education, where the basics of a foreign language may be learned in an incredibly short time.)

What this means in practical terms is that you can, once you begin to become familiar with this territory, begin to exploit it in a number of ways (see the next chapter, Chapter 14, "The Power of Affirmations").

There is yet another way this relaxed, though conscious, state can be utilized. It relates to the next type of sleep.

## THE DREAM STATE

Every sensory experience you have, everything you see, touch, hear, taste, and smell from the moment you awaken, is recorded in your brain. In fact, this has been happening on a daily basis since before you were born. Each experience has a loading—an emotional or intellectual charge—that invests it with more or less significance on the subconscious level. During much, but not all, of the dream state, your mind processes the events and enacts its own seemingly illogical, and largely symbolic, regimen of stress management. It is absolutely essential that this happen for our health and sanity. If we are deprived of this safety valve, we quickly become dysfunctional.

We all must and all do dream, even if we remember nothing of it. For the most part, our dreaming is chaotic, random, fragmented, and non-sequential. In other words, it is inefficient.

## DEEP, DREAMLESS SLEEP

Deep, dreamless sleep is the most valuable aspect of sleep for physical and mental restoration and repair. Each person's need for this is quantitatively different, depending on age and the impact of the day's activities on your body and mind. Also, the amount of time spent in this restorative state is influenced by the time we spend dreaming. To efficiently use the time we have available for deep rest, it is essential to maximize it by spending less time in the dream process.

It is possible to structure and program the dream state so we move through this necessary period of subconscious stress management more swiftly and efficiently, thereby making more time available for the natural restorative processes of deep sleep. The key to this positive alteration of dreaming pattern is in the technique of Unwinding.

THE PRACTICE IS SIMPLE, easy, and much like running a video backwards with your finger occasionally on the "pause" button. When you relax in bed and reach the point of sleep, just before you drop off, mentally travel back through the day three times. Each of the three journeys only takes a few moments, and each is subtly different. It is not important whether you visualize clearly, or simply recall the events in word sequences.

> **MASTERY SOLUTIONS IN PRACTICE:**
>
> **Unwinding**

### First journey

Take your awareness back to the evening mealtime. Recall the meal: who was there, what was said and done, what you wore, what you ate. Then go back to mid-afternoon. Recall the afternoon: where you were, who was there, what you did. Then return to mid-day, or lunchtime; repeat the exercise. Go back to mid-morning; repeat. Finally recall the moment you were first aware that you were awake.

### Second Journey

Repeat the process, but this time use those general segments of the day as signposts only and don't pause for long. Fill in the intervening periods with as much detail as you can recall, but don't dwell on any particular incident. Move more quickly than in the first journey.

### Third Journey

Move very swiftly and as comprehensively as you can, back through the entire waking period. Let the entire practice suddenly, emphatically, drop. Become aware, in a very relaxed way, of the rhythm of your breathing. Mentally count the breath backwards from 100.

## SLEEP EFFICIENCY

When you awaken in the morning, you ought to feel restored and refreshed, ready to take on whatever challenges the day might bring. Whether or not you do feel that way depends, apart from your general level of health and vitality, on the efficiency of your sleep.

The Unwinding technique is an ideal preparation for efficient and more valuable sleep. If it is combined with other practices such as "Steady Gazing" (see Practice 2, page 137), its effects can be enhanced.

You may not leap out of bed the morning after you use the technique for the very first time, but if you incorporate it into your routine, you will quickly begin to feel its benefits.

## DEALING WITH INSOMNIA

There are many levels of insomnia. If you have difficulty in getting to sleep; if your sleeping pattern is irregular; if you awaken frequently; if your sleep is too easily broken by minor disturbances; or if there is simply not enough of it and it does not provide enough restoration of energy, you experience insomnia.

Insomnia can be both a cause and a symptom of stress. When it persists it can severely impair performance. The stress that comes from the difficulties involved in trying to function effectively with reduced reserves of energy as a result of insomnia can cause more insomnia (as can worrying about insomnia itself!).

A stimulant lifestyle is one of the major contributors to insomnia. Under its broad heading are aspects of modern life such as:

### Beverages

Including not only the obvious ones like tea and coffee but also "soft" drinks that contain caffeine and high concentrations of sugar. Caffeine is a diuretic, which means that you are more likely to have to break your sleep period to go to the toilet. Alcohol, which can be dehydrating, can also adversely affect your sleep.

### TV News and Programming, Videos, and Movies

The emotional and mental involvement with these dramas as they unfold on the small or large screen can cause elevated levels of stress chemicals to be present in the bloodstream. Make sure you don't view them too soon before bedtime.

If you are concerned that insomnia may be a serious problem, it's advisable to consult your doctor. It is, however, best not to resort to medication without first exploring, with the help of your physician, the many other helpful, natural processes to aid sleep.

Ironically, many prescription medications for insomnia actually interfere with or suppress the dreaming phase of sleep and hamper the natural stress management processes during this phase.

## AIDS TO SLEEP; HELP FOR INSOMNIA

There are many other factors that can affect the quality and quantity of the rest and the sleep you enjoy, and one of the most important is regular, gradual exercise (see also Chapter 6, "Holistic Health," page 54). Exercise in the evening should, however, not be done too close to bedtime. You will also derive more benefit if it's performed either on an empty stomach or at least two hours after a meal.

What, when, and how much you eat during your evening meal will also have a great bearing on how you sleep. You will have to determine for yourself, by experience and experimentation, the food composition and quantity that best suits your individual sleep requirements. Some people sleep superbly after a heavy meal, others after a light one.

Regularity of routine is one of the most significant factors in establishing a wholesome sleep pattern. Your body becomes easily habituated to an established order and sequence of daily events, as does your mind.

The old adage that an hour of sleep before midnight is worth two after that time is especially true in terms of the body's natural, cir-cadian rhythm. Irregular periods of exposure to variable intensities of light disrupt the function of the brain's master gland, the *pituitary*, together with its minor but still important partner, the *pineal gland*. All of the secretions of the endocrine (hormone-secreting) glands are, in turn, affected.

We have liberated ourselves, as a species, from the limitations of available light (the sun) but we have sacrificed much of our health and vitality to the "tyranny" of the electric light bulb. I'm not advising that you should go to bed as soon as it becomes dark outside, but suggest you strive for your own personal balance in terms of exposure to artificial light. If you make positive adjustments, you will notice the difference!

# CHAPTER 14

# The Power of Affirmations

"AFFIRMATIONS" HAVE BEEN A pow-
erful feature of personal development for the past decade. These are
short, positive statements aimed at altering both your self-concept
and your perceived relationship to the world. In principle, its effectiveness depends on regular repetition, becoming, in fact, a form of
positive conditioning.

We all use affirmations unconsciously when we think or say persistent beliefs to ourselves. Some of these are positive, but many are
not. "I can't remember names" is just a way of telling yourself not
to remember any names. Negative self-image, the perception of
oneself as powerless, ill, or unloved, is usually the result of long-
term conditioning within family or society and can be an effective
form of self-sabotage.

Whatever projects you undertake, or relationships you form, are
undermined by the expectations that persist as a result of these perceptions. A small setback, which would be seen in another perspective by one with a positive self-image, will be blown out of
proportion by negative expectation and will be seen as a confirma-
tion of the self-concept as being "unworthy" or "a failure."

One view of the mind, in simplistic terms (which is, in reality,
not a "thing" but a *living process*), is to compare it to an iceberg.

Only a very small proportion of the iceberg's mass is visible above the water level (this represents the conscious mind) while the greater part is submerged (the subconscious). The far greater potential rests with the hidden area.

Since before birth, your senses have been processing, classifying, prioritizing and storing the information they receive from your environment. Your capacity to classify and interpret your life's events, based on preceding input, increases with each passing year of infancy, childhood, and eventually into adult life.

The nature of your subconscious mind, its structure and the methods by which it processes the information, and your interaction with others became progressively established. This has taken a long time and it is a very individual and complex system, with vast and powerful associations and intricate cross-references.

Your performance and relationships can be severely affected by this deep and potent aspect. The problem lies in the lack of communication between the two levels, and the reality that they are often at cross purposes.

For example, let's say you have a deep and abiding passion for chocolate cake, but on your doctor's advice, you have emphatically decided to eliminate it from your diet. "I will not eat chocolate cake" is a statement and a resolution you make with your conscious mind, and you do it quite well, consciously avoiding every temptation to eat chocolate cake. At a party, you have a wonderfully interesting conversation with an inspiring and stimulating person, and in the middle of the conversation, the host comes to you with a silver platter of exquisite chocolate cakes. You extend your hand and the cake is in your mouth before you can blink an eye. This is the subconscious at work. It has taken advantage of your distracted conscious mind and managed to do just what it wanted.

Although your conscious decision has been firm and resolute, the subconscious has the power to instantly blow it away. This is a very simplistic example but the principle applies to all dimensions of our lives. The two aspects of mind are not in agreement. What is necessary is to establish a channel of communication which can get both areas focused on the same goal. If you can harness the power of

the subconscious mind and align that power with conscious positivity, you can accomplish anything!

Affirmation is an imposition of the conscious on the subconscious. It is a well-meaning attempt to get this hidden potential "on
side," and often produces short-term results but it is a bit like trying
to wear down Mt. Everest with a silk scarf! It can be done, maybe,
but it's not a task you would reasonably expect to accomplish within
a year. It is as if there is a doorway between the two dimensions of
mind, conscious and subconscious. There needs to be, otherwise
our thinking would be swamped by the vast subconscious. To effectively communicate from conscious to subconscious, we need to be
able to open that doorway sufficiently to allow our new and positive
suggestion to slip through and take hold.

In the previous chapter some mention was made of the opportunity presented by the "borderline state" for implanting both information and positive directives. If you can enter and prolong your
stay in this state, your chances of positively influencing the subconscious mind are greatly enhanced. In the borderline state, it is as if
the doorkeeper between the two levels of mind gets drowsy and
relaxed, making it possible to slip a suggestion past this sentry. It
takes *just once* for the subconscious to accept the suggestion, and
you will have both levels working together for a common goal. It
may not take place the first or even the tenth time you use the
method, but with perseverance, it will happen.

It is definitely a thousand times more effective and likely to produce deep and permanent change than standing in front of your
mirror in the morning and repeating "I love you" or "I am powerful"
to your reflection. If you are already using affirmations, or would
like to use them more effectively, it's best to use them during your
practice of Conscious Relaxation. The next best time is while you
are on the threshold of sleep.

The vast potential of combining affirmations with the borderline
state can be applied to many aspects of your life, but it is more
appropriate to settle on a single resolution and deal with that first
before moving on to other aspects. It may be that you want to
address some habit or aspect of your personality that you recognize

as hampering your full expression of life or it may be that you want to reverse some current illness or disease. When you decide on the most important topic for you, keep the expression positive, such as "I will" or "I am" rather than "I will not."

Other crucial aspects include:

*Your own* personal language, phrasing, and emphasis is much more effective than any you can get from a book or a tape. The way you speak to yourself must be easily recognized by your subconscious. It may be more appropriate for you to say, "I'm a really marvelous person" than "I am a warm, loving human being."

It is also best to establish a regularity, a routine time and place. Keep your phrasing unchanged, until you feel you have achieved the desired result.

# CHAPTER 15

## Stress Management Routines

IF YOU SUFFER FROM stress (and this includes everyone now living in our technological society), it follows that you will have to make alterations to your lifestyle. This is especially so if you want not simply to survive, but to perform optimally at work and get the most enjoyment from your personal life.

Depending on the degree stress affects your life, those alterations may have to be major. But before you map out a comprehensive program for yourself, there is one thing that you really have to understand. Embarking on this journey of empowerment through stress management, any change—even the most powerfully positive change—is in itself *another* stress factor.

Any changes should be gradual and progressive. Make sure that each element of your program is approached rationally and with as little disruption to your routine as possible. There is no competition in this game, especially with yourself. High achievers: *please understand this principle thoroughly*. The more slowly and gently you approach your mastery of stress, the better your results will be.

You also need to appreciate that the program you are initiating is not a short-term fix. Look at it from the long-range planning point of view. It is a life-long process, and not an event or finite goal. If you are serious about living all aspects of your life to the full, it will become a natural part of your lifestyle until the day you die. The stress and the challenges *will never decrease*. What changes is how you will *encounter* that stress and those challenges.

## JUST LIKE BRUSHING YOUR TEETH: THE SIX EVENTS

Even with the most flexible (or chaotic) daily schedule or routine, you can choose up to six events or moments that regularly recur. For example, these things can be turning the key in the ignition of your car, pulling into the parking lot, going up in an elevator, eating lunch, buying your evening paper, and turning the key in the door back at home.

The secret to success in stress mastery is to take any one of the techniques you find valuable (it may be the Centering Breath or Body Check) and practice it for a fixed period that you can easily accommodate. For example, you may decide to practice the Centering Breath from the time you turn the key in the ignition until you reach your first or second traffic light. The techniques may vary at different times of the day, depending on your situation. There is one criterion: the method should not interfere with the activity you are engaged in, but preferably enhance it.

The value of this approach lies in *painless reprogramming*: the new is slipped in alongside, or added to, the existing, unconsciously accepted sequence of events. When you do this, you defuse the negative impact of change and start to feel the benefits immediately. The aim is to make the process as ordinary and natural as brushing your teeth.

The experience of the positively altered states of body and mind for brief periods throughout your working day prevents the otherwise unmitigated buildup of stress. You counteract the stress *as it happens*, rather than carry an ever-increasing load.

For most people, cumulative stress is not dealt with until the time of their annual vacation. Apart from the stresses of organizing, packing, and traveling, it takes most of the vacation time to even begin to unwind and enjoy the holiday. By the time you settle into a new relaxed rhythm, the thought of returning to work is already lurking, causing the old stress to resurface.

## THE MINI-VACATION: A HOLIDAY EVERY DAY

Although using the six events is a method for preventing cumulative stress, it's also a bit like swimming in the ocean of stress and using the techniques to help you keep at least one nostril above water. To optimize work and personal performance, however, at least once a day you need to completely and utterly get out of the ocean and onto dry land—shake off the residual drops and take a real rest on the beach. The passport to this mini-vacation is the technique of Conscious Relaxation. The benefits of this state are fully described in Chapter 5, "An Antidote for Stress" and the method itself is in Practice 9, page 179.

Apart from deep and valuable physical, mental, and emotional rest and restoration, this state also provides the opportunity to explore, through the processes of creative visualization, your vast and dormant creative potential. Through regular, daily practice of this technique, you not only get out onto the beach for a rest, but when you return to the ocean, you can swim in it with enjoyment and purpose, through increased reserves of energy on all levels.

Although Conscious Relaxation demands some time (no less than twenty minutes), and thus may seem to contradict the approach of not interfering too much with your established routine, it is so enjoyable and productive that I have included it in these routines.

## PHYSICAL DISCHARGE

The process of physical discharge of stress chemicals is more fully covered in the "Mastery Solutions in Practice" section of Chapter 6, "Holistic Health," but some points need to be reiterated here.

It is absolutely essential that you incorporate *enjoyable* aerobic exercise into your daily routine. This may mean membership in a convenient gym, where circuit training is the best option. Often the feelings of vitality and potency (taking control of your well-being not the least) provide sufficient positive reward and reinforcement to sustain an ongoing program. Be careful not to become competitive with yourself. Stay friendly with yourself and remember that it is more important to establish regularity than to achieve short-term goals. Keep the weight down and the regularity up. Take the stairs and not the elevator whenever time permits.

Use the incredibly powerful "Camel" (see Practice 6, page 160). This has a specific focus on the largest and most powerful body muscles and can superbly discharge levels of stress in a very short time.

Establish the Airlock routine (see "Mastery Solutions in Practice," Chapter 12). Don't forget to negotiate your needs with your partner and your family.

# YOGA PRACTICES

# An Introduction

THE BEGINNINGS OF YOGA are lost in the mists of time, but it is most certainly not exclusively Hindu, or even Indian in origin. I have seen firsthand evidence of classical yoga practice in the statuary of San Augustin in Colombia, South America. Archeologists describe the "contortions" and postures depicted there as some sort of esoteric gymnastics. But to the initiated eye, many are perfect representations of complex classical yoga postures that require much training and dedication to master.

It seems that yoga was once a worldwide culture, as supporting archeological evidence has been reported in such diverse locations as southern France, Scandinavia, and Egypt. It is probable that it was mostly lost during periods of geographical and political upheaval. It was, fortunately, preserved intact in India over millennia, and came to be woven into the fabric of Indian culture.

Yoga is, emphatically, *neither a religion nor Indian!* Although we can be grateful to the generations of Indian practitioners who have experimented on themselves, passed on the results of those experiments and thereby enriched the body of demonstrated theory, it's more important that this experiential knowledge is now available to us.

Unfortunately, yoga has often been "packaged" to the West in partial, fragmented presentations, and has been frequently associated with various quasi-religious cults and sects. This has really been a disservice both to yoga and to potential practitioners. Now, there is an enormous body of hard scientific research both completed and in progress all over the world, which is effectively demonstrating the vast potential of this truly "human" science. Central to the science is the existence of a "life force," a coordinating and cohesive energy that flows in predetermined pathways through our body. Called *prana,* it's a bioelectrical substratum or energy framework that the body's health and vitality depends on. Early maps, or depictions, of this flow of energy were taken from India into China, and it was in correspondence with these depictions that the science of acupuncture was refined. In acupuncture, the very same energy is called *chi* or *k'i.*

All yoga practices aim at harmonizing and balancing this flow of energy. They use static and dynamic postures, subtle and potent breathing techniques and disciplines of concentration and meditation to achieve this.

The physical postures are *not* simply exercises. They are meant to achieve deep equilibrium in the organic function of the various body systems. Your skeletal, muscular, circulatory, respiratory, digestive, nervous, and hormonal systems are all positively affected by them.

The breathing techniques do *not* simply promote efficient respiration. They are a pathway to exploring and establishing great control over our inner climate, in physiological, mental, and emotional terms. They also aim to increase the overall quantity and quality of energy and vitality available to us.

The concentration and meditation techniques are not to promote "navel-gazing" or hasten your withdrawal from mainstream life to a remote Himalayan cave. The techniques help you proceed in life with energy, enthusiasm, and intuition and access your deep reserves of creativity, while they provide periods of psychological rest and cellular restoration.

Ultimately, these techniques are the gateway to illuminating your "sleeping city," the vast and as yet dormant areas of your brain. As a species, we are currently using only a small percentage of the brain. On the evolutionary highway, that's like having a reserve fuel tank four times the capacity of the one we're using!

I hope this brief overview dispels any superficial preconceptions you may have had about yoga practice. In this science, *you* are the scientist, and your body and mind are the laboratory. The experiment is YOU. Approach it slowly and gently with friendliness at all times. If some aspect of practice doesn't agree with you—reject it.

Together with instruction in each of the practices, a basic outline is provided, suggestions for applying the techniques and their benefits. It is important also for you to understand and appreciate the rationale intellectually, so that you can proceed with confidence and enthusiasm.

## PRACTICE 1

# Shaking All Over &
# The Child Pose

THIS IS THE FASTEST and most effective warm-up technique I know, creating heat and bringing blood swiftly to the areas concentrated on. When you are extremely cold, you shiver. This is the body's natural attempt to produce warmth through vibration and movement. In Shaking All Over, this approach is amplified and applied, specifically and systematically, to all the major joints of your body. It should be used before any form of physical exercise and can also be applied regularly if you are in a sedentary occupation.

## SHAKING ALL OVER

### Feet and Ankles

Take a relaxed stance. Transfer all your weight onto your left leg. Extend your right, straightened leg slightly out to your side, allowing your foot and ankle to totally relax. Make rapid movements with the straight leg, so that the foot moves very rapidly. Continue for about ten seconds, then change legs and repeat.

### Knees and Thighs

From a relaxed stance, keep your feet in contact with the floor, and bend each knee in turn so that the action of bending your knee raises your heel only. Your toes and the balls of your feet remain in contact with the floor. Make the movement as fast as you can while allowing the thighs and knees to shake loosely and rapidly. Most of the action should be felt in the large thigh muscles (quadriceps) and the knee joints. The hamstrings at the back of the thighs are also involved. Maintain about ten seconds of rapid movement.

### Pelvis, Buttocks and Lower Back

Slightly bend your knees in the stance. Bend your arms, tucking your elbows and inner sides of your upper arms against your ribcage. Clench your fists, thumbs uppermost, and begin to make short, fast, punching movements with the forearms, transferring the movement that is created to your buttocks and lower back. The trick is to keep your buttocks loose. Once you have established the rhythmic, rapid movement (somewhere between the "shimmy" and the "twist"), you can experiment with stretching the lower back while doing it.

### Wrists, Elbows and Shoulders

Allow your hands and fingers to hang loosely at the ends of your arms, by your sides, then shake your arms and hands rapidly, alternating between up and down and sideways movements at your wrists. Continue the movements up to your elbows, bringing in a rapid partial rotation of your forearms. Slowly raise your arms out to your sides while continuing the movement, allowing the whole arm to shake vigorously, and feel this at your shoulder joints.

### Head and Neck

Keep your facial muscles relaxed and mouth partially open. Begin making rapid but very small movements in your neck. The object here is not to throw the head from side to side, but to set up a rapid vibration. Keep the mouth partially open so that the cheeks and lips participate in the movement.

This completes the Shaking All Over series. Run through your whole body as many times as you feel necessary, emphasizing those areas that require extra attention.

## THE CHILD POSE

In this posture, we see that the lumbar spine is gently stretched, the abdomen is compressed against the thighs and its movement restrained, while the head is moderately lowered, allowing gravity to assist blood flow from the heart to the brain.

There are major constrictions in the legs, both at the knees and at the hips. These constrictions considerably reduce the quantity of blood available to your legs, and thereby increase the volume available to the upper portion of your body, including your abdomen, chest, and head.

It is worth noting that in this posture, the large muscles of the thighs (the body's major consumers of blood) are largely removed from the circulatory equation. Effectively, the work of the circulatory system has been reduced by about a third.

The major portion of blood volume is retained in the upper two-thirds of the body, where all the vital organs are situated, including the brain. As respiration proceeds at a very efficient level during the practice, energizing the blood and removing waste gases, a situation develops in which the actual quality and quantity of the blood available to these vital organs is significantly improved.

We now introduce a very dynamic phenomenon: the natural process of breathing. First, we need to examine the body's trunk. This area, from the pelvis to the neck, is basically a hollow barrel, containing all the important life-preserving organs. It is divided into two chambers: the upper portion contains the heart and lungs, and the lower half, the organs of digestion and reproduction. What divides these two chambers is the sheet of muscle called the diaphragm. For our examination, the trunk can be likened to a bicycle pump. The diaphragm is the plunger and the trunk is the barrel of the pump.

This plunger is in constant motion as we breathe. With each inhalation, it flattens downward, creating positive pressure in the

lower chamber and compressing the contents of the abdominal cavity. At the same time, negative pressure (partial vacuum) is created
in the thoracic chamber, allowing air, under atmospheric pressure,
to flow into the lungs.

Under normal circumstances, the positive pressure in the abdominal cavity would be relieved by an expansion of the belly. If you
watch a baby breathing, the only movement seems to be the rise
and fall of her belly. In the Child Pose, however, the abdominal wall
is restrained by the thighs and not permitted to expand. This con-
verts the automatic breathing process into a dynamic, compressive
massage of the abdominal contents.

Each time you breathe in, the amplified pressure is applied to the
internal organs, creating a slow rhythmic massage of the liver, pancreas, spleen, kidneys and supra renal glands, uterus and ovaries or
prostate gland, together with the entire lower digestive tract.

The effect of this massage is much deeper than can ever be provided by any external masseur. Blood, of much higher quality than
would normally be available, is systematically rinsed through these
major organs. Toxins and metabolic byproducts are flushed out and
the organs are revitalized.

Finally, because of the gentle downward inclination of the head,
the work of your heart in supplying blood to the brain is eased by
gravity. The brain itself, and particularly the pituitary gland (the
master gland controlling hormone secretion), is supplied with this
same high-quality blood. The process of respiration becomes progressively more efficient as the posture is prolonged, with the rate of
respiration gradually decreasing in response to effective carbon
dioxide ($CO_2$) elimination. This creates a state of chemical and
hormonal equanimity.

It does take some time to establish the internal dynamic which
makes all these factors work together to produce the result. You
don't really begin to experience the benefits until you hold the posture for at least five minutes. The more time you spend in the pose,
the more valuable it becomes.

## The Practice

Starting from a comfortable kneeling position, clasp one wrist behind your back with your other hand. Tilt your head slightly up and back, with your eyes looking up towards your forehead. Inhale moderately deeply. Then, while exhaling, bend forward from your waist, keeping your spine straight, with your head slightly back, to eventually bring your belly into contact with your thighs.

At the end of the forward movement, relax your head and neck, resting your forehead on the floor. You may either keep your hands behind your back (which will augment the effect of gravity on blood flow to your brain), or release them and allow your arms to rest relaxed by your sides, the backs of your hands touching the floor.

Once you assume the pose and make any adjustments for your comfort, bring your awareness to your natural breathing process, and to the pressure alternately applied and relieved by the expansion and contraction of your belly against your thighs. It sometimes helps to mentally repeat, "I know I'm breathing in, I know I'm breathing out," and to count the breaths in this way, backward from a predetermined number.

## Releasing the Pose

When you are ready, stretch your arms forward, bringing your palms down onto the floor. Rise slowly, straightening your arms, and rock

Practice 1A

*The Child Pose*

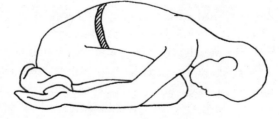

forward onto your hands and knees. Keep your head relaxed. Remain like this for a few moments. Then, gently raise your head while depressing your lower back as you breathe in. Let your head come down slowly and gently as you arch your back, breathing out. Repeat this gentle movement a few times.

### Duration
Be guided by your own direct experience. Although the beneficial minimum may be five minutes, you can slowly work up to this by starting with one minute, over a period of several weeks. Add a few seconds each day.

### Variations According to Physical Limitations
Many people whose lives are mainly sedentary will find some difficulties in assuming the complete posture. If you are not very flexible in the knees or ankles, are somewhat overweight, or suffer from high blood pressure, there are some adaptations that can make the Child Pose more comfortable, at least in the early stages.

In the case of hypertension, or lack of flexibility in the spine, raise your forehead or support it with several pillows or towels. This reduces the flow of blood to your head and eases the amount of forward bending, especially in your lower back. If you are overweight, your knees and thighs can be separated to relieve discomfort. If there is discomfort at your knees, ankles or instep, this can be relieved by placing folded towels at these areas.

### Benefits
The Child Pose is particularly effective in cases of asthma and chronic bronchitis, because of its regulatory effect on the adrenal cortex. It can also be an important part of relieving constipation, as well as generally strengthening your immune system.

My personal experience with this technique allows me to recommend it wholeheartedly for depression. In the period following my wife's death, it was incredibly useful. Any extreme emotional state—such as anger, anxiety, depression or fear—causes a chemical and hormonal imbalance. This practice, while it does nothing about whatever may be causing the emotional crisis, restores biochemical equanimity. Before you can do anything about the cause of such a state, you first need to get out of it!

# PRACTICE 2

# Steady Gazing

IN 1978, WHILE TEACHING general yoga and meditation classes at the Perth YMCA in Western Australia, one of my students, a woman in her mid-fifties, asked if she could consult with me to see if yoga could help with a problem she described as "insomnia." Her physician had recommended she attend yoga classes, as medication had not relieved it. She had a strong fundamentalist Christian background and, were it not for her doctor's recommendation and the fact that my classes were conducted under the auspices of the YMCA, would never have attended. Her religious background misinformed her that yoga was "the work of the devil" and "a heathen religion."

I observed her progress throughout most of the first term and was pleased with the obvious effort she made. I often spoke of yoga's specific therapeutic applications, and after a class toward the end of the term, she approached me personally. We made an appointment for her to come to my Centre.

On the appointed day she duly arrived; it had taken considerable courage for her to personally approach me, and even more to actually come to my Centre. It was only the personal confidence she had established with me in the class situation and her desperate need for relief that allowed her to override her negative conditioning.

She related to me her malady. Every morning at around 2 A.M. she awoke in mortal terror. She felt she was being crushed, and couldn't breathe. She would then lie in bed, paralyzed by this nameless terror and unable to sleep until it was time for her to get up and get ready for work. She would delay going to bed, in order to make herself as tired as possible, but to no avail. She lived in fear of going to sleep, as the terror was unbearable. This had been going on for almost twenty years!

I immediately thought of the meditative technique of Inner Silence. I was on the point of giving her preliminary instruction in this method when, intuitively, the practice of Steady Gazing came to mind. I reasoned that it would better help to "clear the deck" before proceeding with the deeper practice. I instructed her immediately in the practice of Steady Gazing and asked her to practice it daily, immediately before retiring to bed, for a period of fifteen days. We then arranged that she would return for monitoring and further instruction.

After a couple of weeks, she telephoned and asked if she could see me again. Thinking that the period specified for the Steady Gazing had elapsed and that she would then be ready for the Inner Silence, we made the appointment.

When she arrived, I was pleasantly surprised by nothing less than a transformation in her appearance. She looked years younger, had lost the haunted, exhausted demeanor of the previous interview, and seemed very relaxed. She told me about her practice of Steady Gazing.

On the first night, she had performed the technique as instructed immediately before going to bed. There was no change in her sleeping pattern. She still awoke at the same time, with the attendant fear. This was repeated on the second night also. On the third night she awoke again, but with a perfectly clear and detailed recollection of the original event that lay at the source of her problem.

Twenty years previously, she had been married to a disturbed man. She had at various times been sexually, verbally and physically abused by him. Eventually, they separated.

On the night her terror began, he gave her a narcotic, which rendered her helpless while he and a group of his friends repeatedly raped and abused her. In her narcotic state, she had been completely aware of every detail of the experience, but totally vulnerable and powerless. It had been so horrific that she completely suppressed it.

When she totally recalled the memory, she broke down and cried until dawn. Then she got up and went to work as usual. The following evening she practiced Steady Gazing again before bedtime. She felt that she should continue to see if there was any more to be released. The next morning she was late for work for the first time in many years. She slept without interruption, and didn't even hear her alarm clock ringing!

For the next seven days, she continued with the practice and then decided to try sleeping without Steady Gazing. Her healthy sleeping pattern continued. When she had related this account, she thanked me for my help, informed me that she didn't feel as if she needed any more yoga, and left. I never saw her again.

### The Practice

Steady Gazing, one of the six "cleansing" practices that constitutes classical Hatha yoga, consists of steady relaxed gazing at a single focal point. The object used should be at eye level, central, and at arm's length. You can practice on a candle flame; a black dot on a white background (or chromatic variations); a crystal, yantra, mandala; or the reflection of your own face in a mirror. However, for general purposes, the candle flame is by far the most suitable and safe. To use the other objects, I strongly recommend that you seek the guidance of a competent yoga instructor.

**Phase One:** With the candle set up as indicated, sit, with your eyes closed, in a comfortable and steady position that you will be able to maintain for some time. First, keep your body still. This is in itself a potent meditative technique, helping you become intensely aware, moment to moment, of establishing and maintaining stillness throughout your entire body.

After a while, open the eyes and begin to gaze at the tip of the wick. This should be relaxed and steady. Do not force concentration or tense your eyes. Your awareness during this period should keep to the thought, "I am gazing at the candle flame—I am gazing at the candle flame." In effect, you are bringing your awareness constantly and repeatedly to what you are doing.

When your eyes become too uncomfortable and begin to water, gently close them. With regular practice, you will find that you can keep your eyes open for longer periods without discomfort. It is essential that there be absolutely no physical movement during Phase One.

**Phase Two:** Having closed your eyes, become aware of any after-images that may appear. In just the same relaxed way as when your eyes were open, continue to gaze, behind your closed lids, at whatever you may see.

Note any changes in color or form and allow the image to remain steady. It should not dance around. If this does happen (the after-image can often be very unstable in the early stages of practice), consciously relax your eyes, and the image will still itself proportionately.

When the after-image has disappeared completely, this is the end of Phase Two, and constitutes one round of the practice. At this point you may either end the practice or continue alternating the phases according to experience, comfort, and time available.

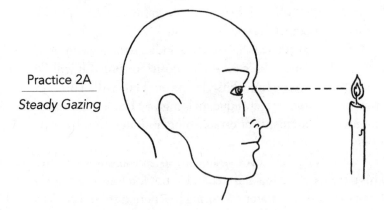

Practice 2A

*Steady Gazing*

## Extended and Deeper Practice

If you find that you really enjoy the technique and would like to do more rounds, these guidelines may be helpful:

**Round One:** Same as above.

**Round Two:** As soon as you open your eyes again to continue, proceed exactly as you did in the first round, but mentally establish a connection with the flame. Cultivate the feeling that you are absorbing, through this connection, the positive qualities that humanity has associated with the candle flame over the centuries: brightness, warmth, honesty—the purifying aspect of the fire element. In Phase Two of this round, continue this process with the after-image.

**Round Three:** Upon opening your eyes, immediately become aware of:

1. *Your Visual Field:* The candle and flame.

2. *Your Medium of Perception:* The faculty of sight, your eyes themselves, through which you are looking out at the visual field.

3. *Yourself:* You who are looking out through the eyes at the visual field. You can call this "I, Myself, or Self."

Rotate your consciousness among these three components, mentally repeating or being aware: "Candle flame, my eyes (feel your eyes in their sockets)—self." Your awareness rests briefly on each component in turn, creating a sense of mental movement inward. After a while, change the direction of this rotation to outward: "Self, eyes, flame." You can play with the method, changing speed and direction as you choose, until you close your eyes and begin Phase Two.

In Phase Two, cultivate the feeling and the experience of drawing the after-image inward from its position in front of your closed eyes towards the center of your brain.

## Background of the Practice

Each of your senses is a door, through which your consciousness is connected to the world. Each sense has its own specific reservoir of energy, and each sense has its own memory. In the case of sight, every visual experience you have ever had is recorded, from your birth to the moment you're reading this.

Throughout your waking hours, your eyes are in a process of constant motion and internal muscular activity as the focal length continuously adapts. They are also subject to varying intensities of light as you turn your head. Often the light input will be vastly different for each eye.

During this practice, however, the eyes are perfectly still and relaxed. The light intensity remains constant and the input is exactly the same for both eyes. This brings about habituation and subsequent relaxation in the visual cortex on both sides of the brain. Gradually, the eyes become more still, and simultaneously, the turbulence of your mind reduces as your concentration increases.

## Benefits

Steady gazing is a powerful tool for developing concentration and helps with nearsightedness. In conjunction with the practice of "Unwinding," it can also positively influence sleeping patterns, helping you to awaken refreshed and restored.

Even practiced for brief periods, it can help to establish balance to the whole nervous system. With extended practice, it can be a gateway to your creativity and intuition.

# Brain Massage &
# The Humming Bee

EVERYONE THINKS OF THE brain as a fixed organ, unmoving within the bony protective structure of the skull. The reality is that it does move, in a rhythmic way, swelling and contracting in time with your breath. It responds to changing blood volume. With the following technique, this natural phenomenon is amplified by emphasizing your exhalation.

## BRAIN MASSAGE

Sitting with your spine comfortably erect, close your eyes and relax for a few moments. Inhale through your nose, comfortably and evenly.

Keeping your mouth closed, exhale through your nose with a short, sharp expulsion. The shortness and sharpness of this expulsion is the most important aspect of the practice and is amplified by a swift and pronounced contraction of your belly muscles. This constitutes one breath.

Allow your belly muscles to immediately relax and inhale again, effortlessly, followed by a short, sharp exhalation. Throughout the process, the conscious emphasis is always on the exhalation. Inhalation should be automatic and almost unconscious. It takes care of itself as the exhalation punctuates and establishes a comfortable rhythm.

Perform one round of seven to ten breaths.

### Important

After the last exhalation of the round, slowly inhale deeply, but not too full. Bend your head forward and tuck your chin into the hollow at the base of your throat (or as close as possible without causing any neck strain). With your hands on your thighs, straighten your arms and raise both shoulders. Hold your breath for a few seconds.

When you are ready to release your breath, follow this sequence exactly: First relax your arms and lower your shoulders. Next, slowly raise your head. Then, before you breathe out, inhale just a little to open the airway. Finally, exhale slowly and evenly. Breathe normally until you feel ready to start another round.

While holding your breath, keep your awareness in the space behind your eyes (in the brain itself).

There should be no dizziness or faintness at any time with this technique. If you experience these symptoms, reduce the number of breaths per round and also reduce the strength of the exhalations. If the feeling persists, do not hold your breath at the end of the round.

Begin with three rounds of up to ten breaths. As you become proficient, gradually increase the number of breaths per round.

### Benefits

Brain Massage breathing does exactly what it says, refreshing your whole brain, especially the frontal lobes of the cerebral cortex. It is a very fast way to restore flagging concentration and interrupt the flow of repetitive, obsessive, or unwelcome thoughts. I often use a limited version (with no breath retention) when I have to drive long distances and begin to lose my concentration.

## THE HUMMING BEE

In 1976 experiments were conducted in Madrid, Spain, to get some idea of the effect of self-generated sound on the human brain. The electrical activity of the brain was monitored in the subjects by electroencephalograph (EEG).

A significant result was that the sound "Mmmmmm," when sustained for some time, produced identical patterns on the EEG to those associated with deep, dreamless sleep. The subjects were very much awake and involved in an activity. Their subjective report was that they felt very calm, relaxed, and centered.

The "Humming Bee" is a breathing technique that utilizes the process of internally generated and specifically directed sound vibration to alleviate anxiety and to reduce cerebral tension (within the brain itself).

Seated comfortably, with your eyes closed, slowly inhale in the Monitoring Breath. Don't overfill your lungs, but rather, feel that the air is gently and purposefully filling a hollow cylinder from your navel to your throat. At the top of the inhalation, gently lower your chin towards your chest and hold your breath for about three seconds.

Raise your head again, take a slight inward breath to open the airway and simultaneously raise your hands, elbows out to your sides, to open the chest. Press the tragus (the small flap of cartilage at the entrance of your ears) gently closed on both ears, using the tips of your index fingers.

Using a controlled exhalation, make a humming sound. This can be as subtle or as loud as your situation and discretion permit. The whole of the exhalation is used to continue this sound, trying to keep it as smooth and uniform in its pitch as you are able. (Find the pitch that feels most comfortable to you.) Before you completely run out of breath, discontinue the sound and lower your hands to your lap.

At this point, when you are beginning the practice, it's fine to take one comfortable normal breath, and then begin again. However, it's ideal to establish a comfortable, controlled rhythm so that the humming sounds are sequential. To do this, it is important not to leave yourself short of breath at the end of the exhalation and also not to inhale too fully. The essence of the technique is to establish the easy rhythm of breathing and a constant, steady, and unwavering sound.

Use the humming sound as a searchlight. Move its focus around inside the head: left side, right side, top, front, back and center. As you do this, your awareness is within the physical brain itself. Find the area in this space that you are most attracted to, and then focus the sound awareness there for the duration of the practice.

## Duration and Frequency

Begin with a regular practice of at least six to ten rounds until the process becomes thoroughly comfortable and you are familiar with the changes in mental state and the general feeling of well-being you produce. The Humming Bee doesn't take very long at all to master and can give profound effects in a short time. When practice has made it fully at your disposal, you can use it at any time.

## Benefits

The soothing action of the sound produces changes in your brain chemistry and in your central nervous system. It can alleviate states of anger and anxiety, and it definitely reduces cerebral tension. It can also help greatly to relieve some types of headache.

# PRACTICE 4

# Joint Rotation

IN 1981, WHILE I operated a yoga center in Adelaide, South Australia, a professional concert pianist came to see me. He was deeply distressed because he had begun to experience diminished flexibility and mobility in his hands and fingers over a period of a few months.

After talking with him for some time, I decided to instruct him in two techniques. The first of these was the practice of joint rotation described here. The second was a specific visualization performed while in the state of Conscious Relaxation.

At the conclusion of our session he offered, in a perfunctory sort of way, to pay me, and I could tell that intellectually, he was not at all satisfied with the practices. I then explained to him the principles of energy flow in the body and finally got him to agree to use the techniques I had shown him for at least one week. I refused to take any money at that point, saying, "Pay me what you think it's worth, when and if it works."

Two days later, he returned with an envelope containing two hundred dollars. He was invigorated and excited at having, as he expressed it, "new hands."

This technique, while physically very gentle, is also very deep and powerful. It consists of a combination of slow controlled movement,

147

breath awareness, sensitization and visualization. Your body joints are structures whose health and unimpaired function your mobility and much of your capacity for enjoyment of life depend on. They are also areas of vulnerability.

Particularly in the modern urban lifestyle, our joints are often not exercised through their full range of movement. As a result, there's a progressive degeneration in the condition of many joints, with conditions such as rheumatism and arthritis common at increasingly earlier stages of life.

In Chinese medicine, toes and fingers relate to the "well" points through which energy enters and leaves acupuncture meridians, while the knees, elbows, ankles, and wrists relate to the "source" points and have a direct bearing on the health of your internal organs. It is at the joints that the balance and flow of prana or "ki" energy may be easily impeded and this can have severe consequences elsewhere in the body.

When purposeful, conscious movement is combined with breath awareness and visualization, the end result is not simply the maintenance or restoration of mobility in the particular joint area, but also and more essentially, the removal of blockages to the flow and balance of this energy.

The technique has been described by Dr. Hiroshi Motoyama, one of the preeminent Japanese researchers in the exploration of the science of acupuncture and the demonstration of the psychophysiological energy flow in the human body, as "acupuncture without needles."

## Movement

In each of the joint areas, from your toes to your head, there is a slow, controlled movement. It consists mainly of rotation, and also flexion and extension. Movements are made in perfect time with your breath. In general terms, inhalation proceeds while the joint structure is moving away from the trunk or the limb it is attached to (an expansive movement) and exhalation takes place as the part moves back towards the body proper (a compressive movement).

### Breathing

The form of breathing used is the Monitoring Breath (see Chapter 8, "The Centering Breath"). Because of its calming and focusing effect, the Monitoring Breath allows you to establish an even and comfortable breathing rhythm while simultaneously enabling you to enter more effectively into the sensitization and visualization aspect of the practice.

### Sensitization

The aim is to bring your awareness totally into the area focussed on. The feeling to be created is that you are actually breathing in and out exclusively through the pores of the skin in the joint concerned.

### Visualization

I am indebted to Marion Wayne (Swami Alokananda Saraswati of Brisbane, Australia) for this visualization. The first couple of movements are performed with your eyes open and gazing intently at the area. You visually impress the image in this way, then close your eyes and visualize the movement as it is being made. Using your imagination, create a greatly magnified view of the skin surface in the area. As you are inhaling, see golden light being drawn in through your pores and bathing the internal structure of the joint. As you exhale on the compressive movement, visualize tiny eruptions, like puffs of dark vapor or smoke, being emitted through the pores.

### Duration and Frequency

The number of rotations is usually ten, but this can be varied up or down according to your personal needs. If your lifestyle is largely sedentary, you are well advised to emphasize your knees and hips. If you spend long periods at a computer keyboard, then fingers, wrists, elbows, shoulders, and neck can also be addressed at regular intervals. This will prevent tension buildup in these areas.

## Benefits

The positive effects of this series are vast. As you bring your mind through the processes of movement, breath awareness, sensitization and visualization to focus on the specific area, so does the flow of energy in the acupuncture meridians adjust and balance itself. This can have a tremendously therapeutic action, not only in the joints in question, but also on major internal organs such as liver, stomach, kidneys, spleen and heart. These all depend for their optimum function on the quality and quantity of life energy (bioelectricity, prana or ch'i) available.

Metabolic by-products, inorganic salts and general accretions that may otherwise limit the range of movement in the joint are gradually released into the blood and lymph and are thereby eliminated from the system. As you age, it is a fact that your enjoyment of life will greatly depend on your mobility. Arthritis and rheumatism do not have to be an inevitable concomitant of the aging process.

Another little realized benefit of the series is a significant increase in fine motor control. As the joints (especially fingers and wrists) are slowly exercised in this deep and comprehensive way, the relevant pathways in the brain in the sensory/motor cortex and cerebellum are strengthened. If you are a musician, brain surgeon, cake decorator, or just simply want to be able to effortlessly pick fleas off your pet dog, this is helpful.

The whole series is a type of active meditation, and generally produces a sense of calm, centering, and well-being. All the practice elements contribute to this effect, especially those processes initiated within the brain itself; that is, the sequential and isolated functions of the motor cortex as each joint or group of joints operates in isolation. This produces a relaxing effect in the cortex *after* each area is operated, much as in Tai Chi, with its slow movement.

Repeat all movements a minimum of six times.

1. **Toe Bending and Separating.** Sit in a comfortable position, with your legs stretched out in front. You may, if you like, support yourself with your hands at your sides on the floor, a little behind your buttocks. Keep your feet still and slowly and gently point your toes down towards the floor, while exhaling in the Monitoring Breath. Be careful not

to use so much force in this movement that you cramp your instep.

Inhale in the same way, while you flex your toes back towards the body and separate them as fully as you can at the end of this movement. Keep your gaze fixed on the toes throughout the first few repetitions, then close your eyes, and enter into the sensitization and visualization process.

2. **Ankle Extension and Flexion:** Keeping your toes relaxed, arch your feet down towards the floor on inhalation, and then back towards you on exhalation.

3. **Ankle Rotation:** As for 1 and 2, but exercising only one side at a time, your heel remains on the floor while the foot sweeps down toward the floor on inhalation and back towards you on exhalation. Rotate each ankle both clockwise and counter-clockwise.

4. **Knee Extension and Flexion:** Clasp your hands under the right thigh, allowing your lower leg to relax, with your knee bent. Slowly straighten your leg as you inhale. At the top of the breath and the end of this straightening movement, flex your foot a little back towards your body and feel the extra movement in your knee joint. As you exhale, bring your thigh back towards your chest and allow your knee to come slowly to the fully bent position, heel near your buttocks. Repeat.

5. **Knee Rotation:** As for step 4, hold your thigh in the same way. Slowly arc a circle with your lower leg around your knee. This joint is not designed for a great amount of rotation, but whatever you can manage will greatly strengthen its ligaments. Inhale as your lower leg sweeps down towards the floor and exhale as it moves upward and over. Rotate in both directions and repeat with the other knee.

6. **Hip Rotation (first variation):** Lie comfortably on your back, with legs stretched out. Raise your right leg, with knee bent, towards your chest. Slowly move the bent leg out to the right and then, while inhaling, straighten your leg and continue the movement out, down then across towards the other leg, so that the heel sweeps close to the

floor. As the leg begins its travel out to the left and up towards the starting position, exhale as your knee slowly bends again. The exhalation continues as the leg describes the upper arc, close to your chest and across and out to the right again. Repeat the as many times as is comfortable, reverse the direction of rotation, then work the other hip in the same way.

Note: This method does not require as much strength in the abdomen as step 7.

7. **Hip Rotation (second variation):** This is the same as step 6 except that your leg is kept straight throughout the movement and your arms are extended at right angles to the trunk, with the backs of your hands maintaining contact with the floor. Make circles as completely as you can. Inhale as your straightened leg sweeps down and across, as far out to the side as possible. Exhale as your leg comes up and over. Reverse the direction of rotation after the appropriate number of rounds, then repeat with your other leg.

Note: This variation is much stronger than the preceding one, particularly with regard to the binding ligaments of the joint, so proceed with caution and only according to your ability. Also, as the leg is at the farthest point of its arc on the opposite side, there is considerable torque to the lumbar/sacral area of your spine. If you are sufficiently relaxed in the movement, you may hear a "clunk" as the lumbar spine adjusts itself.

8. **Spinal Rolls:** This movement is performed slowly, in time with your breath. It is important to perform it on a folded blanket or something similar. In the early stages of your practice, be careful not to roll too far backward, straining your neck. Sitting with your legs outstretched, bend both your knees and draw them up towards your chest. Clasp your hands around your knees or shins, as much as you can comfortably do. Inhale, then as you exhale, roll backward onto your shoulders. Inhale as you roll forward onto your buttocks. Your awareness of breath is located in your spine. As you roll backward, your breath awareness moves from

your sacrum to your base of your neck and, conversely, as you come forward.

This movement not only stimulates the junctions of your spinal column and the nerves that emanate from there, but also gives a wonderful compressive massage to the muscular structures that help to support and maintain the integrity of your spine. Metabolic by-products and residual toxins that may be in your muscle tissue are milked out and disposed of by the circulatory and lymphatic systems.

9. **Finger Extension and Flexion:** Both this and step 10 are performed with both hands simultaneously. Sitting comfortably, extend your arms out in front and focus your gaze on your hands. As you inhale, stretch your fingers apart, in time with your breath, separating them as widely as you can. As you exhale, slowly bend all your fingers, gently bringing your thumbs in, tucking them behind your index and middle fingers while making fists. Repeat.

10. **Wrist Extension and Flexion:** Sitting as for step 9, inhale, slowly bringing your hands down towards the floor. (Keep your hands and fingers straight throughout both phases of the movement.) At the end of this descent, and at the top of your breath, pause for a couple of seconds. Gently bend just your fingertips back towards the undersides of your wrists a few times, feeling the extra extension in your wrist joints as you do this. Exhale while bringing your straightened hands up and back towards your chest. Your awareness is localized in your wrist joints throughout.

11. **Wrist Rotation:** These movements are best performed one wrist at a time. With your right arm outstretched, make a gentle fist with your thumb tucked slightly in. If your thumb is tucked too tightly, you can strain the wrist ligaments. Rotate your wrist first clockwise several times then counterclockwise. Inhale as your fist describes the downward half of the circle and exhale as it moves up and across. Repeat with your other hand. Awareness of your breath is through the pores of your skin at the wrist joint.

12. **Elbow Bending:** Sitting as for step 10, with your hands outstretched but with palms facing upward, inhale, focusing on your elbow joints. Exhale while slowly bending your elbows and bringing your fingertips to your shoulders. As you inhale, slowly straighten your arms and, at the end of the outward movement, move your straightened hands slightly down and out to your sides a little, feeling the extra extension in your elbow joints. The same process can then be repeated with your arms out to your sides.

13. **Shoulder Rotations:** With your fingers resting on your shoulders and your elbows out to your sides, describe full circles with your elbows.

    Exhale as your elbows move upward in front of your chest, bringing them as close to each other as possible during this upward and forward movement. As they separate and move backward, opening out your chest, slowly inhale. After several repetitions, reverse direction.

14. **Neck Rolls:** One of the most tense areas of your body is your neck and shoulders. If this tension is not regularly resolved and becomes chronic, it can structurally affect the cervical vertebrae, the nerves that emanate from the spinal cord in this area, and also circulation to and from the brain. Common end results of unresolved neck tension may be headaches, impaired vision or hearing and also acute pain in the neck itself.

    As your neck is such a delicate and vulnerable structure, it is critical to maintain super-sensitive awareness in preventing injury to this area as you perform the movements.

The Joint Rotation series culminates in this practice. It is the most subtle and slow of all the movements, and it can also swiftly produce a significant and positive alteration of your mental and emotional state when it is performed as a separate technique throughout your day.

Taking even just a few minutes out from a process that may demand unflagging concentration or attention and using this tool can produce a feeling I like to describe as "taking a shower on the inside."

**Note:** The emphasis of breath awareness and visualization, whether you are inhaling or exhaling during any part of the movements involved, can be adjusted according to your preference and whether your focus is desired at the front or at the back of your neck.

If you want to affect the structures at the front of your neck and throat (thyroid and parathyroid glands, larynx and carotid sinus receptors), then inhalation will take place while this area is opened up. Conversely, do this if you are concerned with the muscles at the back of the neck.

**Preparatory Movements:** Any comfortable sitting position that allows your spine to be easily erect is suitable for the neck rolls. There are two sets of movements that should, if time permits, be completed before attempting the full neck rotations. These gently stretch your neck muscles and help to prevent injury or strain.

Slowly exhale a Monitoring Breath, focusing on your neck. Then as you inhale, allow your chin to descend, in time with your breath, towards your chest as far as is comfortable. As you lower your head, become aware of your neck vertebrae opening up, and feel as if you are breathing through the pores of your skin there, drawing in a golden light. As you exhale, raise your head up and back in time with your breath and visualize the eruptions of dark vapor through the pores of your skin as the back of your neck is gently squeezed. Repeat several times. Apply this intensity of visualization particularly in the complete neck rolls.

Next, apply the same process while gently lowering your ear towards each shoulder, breathing in as your head lowers, feeling the opposite side of your neck opening up. Breathe out as your head returns to the central position.

**Complete Neck Rolls:** Begin the full rotation of the neck with the smallest possible circles, gradually increasing the diameter as you expand your comfort zone. The movement, in time with your breath, must be as slow as you can manage. The sensitization and visualization should also be very comprehensive.

Sometimes, because of structural irregularities or tension in your neck musculature, there may be discomfort at certain points of the circle. Proceed slowly, and with such sensitivity that you become aware of these areas before you cause yourself any pain. The moment you become aware of approaching such a restriction, simply raise your head a little, reducing the diameter of the circle at that point to easily pass over the "bump." Usually, by continuing within the above parameters, you will be able to dissolve the tension in your neck.

# PRACTICE 5

# Letting Go

LETTING GO IS ALSO referred to as the "tension relieving" series. It is a very swift and systematic way of resolving accumulated muscular tension. In this practice, all the muscle groups are progressively tightened, then relaxed. The process begins with the feet and legs, and ends with the muscles of your scalp.

As with any exposure to stress, there is a subsequent alteration of your body chemistry. Unless these by-products are discharged (and activity is an effective way of discharging stress chemistry), there are significant changes that occur, biochemically, within your musculature. There is also a corresponding, habituated over-stimulus in the sensory and motor cortex of your brain.

Because each muscle group is worked in isolation from the rest of your body (being alternately contracted and relaxed in sequence), a progressive and very specific journey is made, below the level of consciousness, through the parts of the brain that register sensation from, and control the movement of, these areas. As the muscle groups discharge their stress and relax, so does the brain. You are not only discharging the tension from the muscle group concerned, but also addressing the part of the nervous system that is intimately related to it.

When you begin practicing Letting Go, it can take around twenty minutes to complete the sequence, but with a little regular practice, that time can be reduced to a very efficient six minutes. The ideal time to use the tool is during your "Airlock" procedure at the end of a working day (or while making the transition from one distinct environment to another).

The technique consists of two aspects: contraction and relaxation. The contraction of the muscle group concerned is made gradually and progressively and this action is coordinated with a slow, deep inhalation through your nostrils, using a subtle form of the Monitoring Breath. It takes as long to tighten the muscle as it does to breathe in.

For completely effective practice, it is crucial that the rest of your body remain relaxed as much as possible and uninvolved in the process. While practicing, check from time to time to make sure that you are not tensing your facial muscles (for instance) while you are tensing your leg. It takes a while to acquire the knack. When you reach the top of the inhalation, your breath is held for a count of three while the contraction is maintained at maximum level.

Release of the breath and the accompanying relaxation of the area is totally different from the inhalation and contraction. It is swift and sudden: a matter of instantaneously relinquishing your conscious contraction while allowing the breath to explode through the mouth with the sound "Pah!"

The practice in sequence is fully described in Chapter 12, "Bringing It All Back Home."

# The Thunderbolt Pose

THIS POSTURE IS TRADITIONAL in Japanese Buddhist meditation. Many Westerners initially find it quite uncomfortable, especially in the feet and legs. Its benefits, however, are such that you will find it very worthwhile to persevere with it and gradually extend your capacity to sit in it for a reasonable period of time.

The pose naturally encourages a correct spinal attitude and produces significant changes in the dynamics of blood distribution, which most of its benefits come from. Because less blood gets to the legs, more blood is kept available to the trunk.

The legs, which are major consumers of blood, are largely excluded from the circulatory equation and at the same time the lungs are still functioning efficiently, energizing and removing waste from the fluid. The blood that is then available to the major organs is of a higher quality than normal. This benefit is especially applicable to the digestive process and also to the reproductive organs.

There are also some subtle points, related to the digestive process, which are stimulated by crossing the big toes and pressing the heels to your buttocks.

The Thunderbolt Pose can be ideally used immediately after lunch. It will help efficient assimilation of the food consumed and thereby contribute to better performance in the afternoon. Allow five minutes, minimum, to experience the effects.

## THE CAMEL

Classically, this technique is used to improve posture and help with problems such as constipation. It is important that your stomach be empty, so it is best used before a meal and can be incorporated into your lunchtime regimen.

Although a progression into the pose is given in outline, the first segment is especially beneficial for stress management. In this repeated movement, the quadriceps (muscles of the thighs) are exercised comprehensively. As these muscles are the body's greatest consumers of blood, focusing on them so specifically provides an opportunity for efficient discharge of chemicals in the blood that are the result of stress.

### First Segment

Sitting in the Thunderbolt Pose (see Practice figure 6A), separate your feet. Sit for a few seconds and become aware of your spinal

Practice 6A

*The Thunderbolt Pose (left)*

*Position of feet (right)*

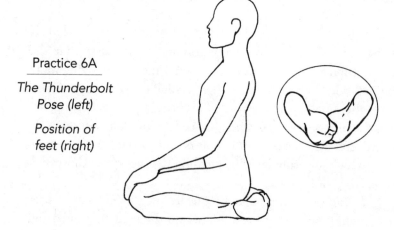

posture, and breathe in the Monitoring Breath. Feel the breath filling your belly and be aware of the subtle sound that allows you to regulate the duration and evenness of your breathing.

As you inhale, rise up to the vertical while simultaneously raising your arms out to your sides until they reach shoulder level. This movement should take as long as the inhalation. As you exhale, slowly lower your arms and return to the starting position.

Repeat the movement according to your fitness. The more slowly you perform it, the stronger the effect in your knee joints, and especially in your thigh muscles. It is better to gradually decrease the speed over days and weeks, strengthening the muscles and the knee ligaments, than to attempt to do it extremely slowly right from the beginning.

## The Classical Practice

Sitting in the Thunderbolt pose, but with the toes tucked under the balls of the feet and the heels raised, proceed as before with the inhalation. When you reach the top of the movement and the breath, slowly exhale while rotating the trunk to the left, reaching down and behind to touch the left heel with the left hand.

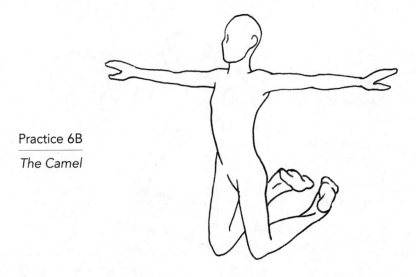

Practice 6B

*The Camel*

Pause for a second, centralizing the trunk in this backward bent attitude with the head allowed to rest back, eyes looking up at the ceiling and with the right arm extended vertically. As you breathe in, release the left hand and rise back to the upright kneeling position. Exhaling, repeat the movement to the right side.

On inhalation, return to the upright, then as you exhale, return to the floor, lowering the arms and thighs in time with the breath. This constitutes one round. Repeat according to your time and fitness. This variation of the Camel is especially good for relieving constipation and for strengthening the lumbar spine.

There is an extension of the practice where, as you reach back, twist a little so that you can reach the opposite heel (that is, left hand on right heel, and conversely). Provided you stay within your comfortable capacity, this applied torque to the spine is also very beneficial. As your comfort zone extends with practice, separate your feet wider to give an extra twist.

Practice 6C

*The Camel:*
*Classical Practice*
*(left)*

*Position of*
*feet (right)*

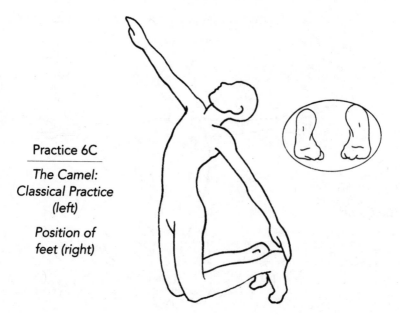

## THE ROARING LION

This is not the sort of technique that you would normally consider using in a public place, unless the mood were too serious and you wanted to provide some entertainment.

It is an ideal preparation for public speaking, or for honing your vocal skills. It removes tension in the throat and frontal lobe of the brain, and can greatly assist in maintaining the general health and resistance to illness in the ears, nose, and throat. It also helps to treat speech impairment. If at all possible, it is a wonderful idea to allow morning sunlight to radiate into the mouth and throat.

Although the following directions are given for the classical pose, don't be daunted if you have difficulty with it. Most of the benefits applicable to stress management can be gained simply by sitting in a chair and following the rest of the instructions.

Sit in the Thunderbolt Pose and separate your knees to more than shoulder-width apart. Lean forward and place the palms of the hands on the floor with your fingers pointing back into, and slightly tucked under, the upper portion of the shins. At this point your elbows should press against the lower sides of the ribcage and the inner forearms are rotated to the front. If you are not sufficiently flexible in the wrists to manage this easily, then make fists of your hands while rotating your forearms and still creating the

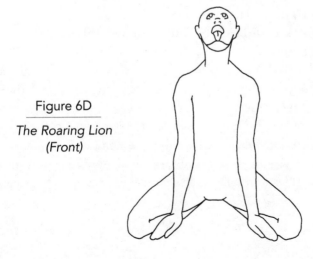

Figure 6D

*The Roaring Lion*
*(Front)*

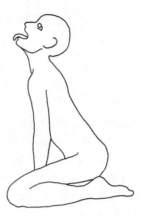

Figure 6E

*The Roaring Lion*
*(Side)*

pressure of the elbows against your ribcage. If this is also too uncomfortable, then allow the fingers to point forward, palms down, keeping the arms locked straight with the inner sides of the elbows against the ribcage.

Inhale through your nose, feeling the air go deep into your belly, as you roll the eyes upward to gaze at the point between your eyebrows. As the eyes move upward, tilt your head back until you feel a roll of gentle pressure at the back of your neck. Open your mouth, extending the tongue out and downward, as if to touch your chin, while tensing the muscles of the front of your neck.

As you exhale, create a prolonged and steady "ah" sound deep in the throat. Adjust the pitch of the sound so that you can feel it predominantly in the larynx. If you are fortunate enough to be able to practice it at dawn, feel the sun's light and warmth entering your mouth and throat.

Don't try to keep going to the point where you are totally out of breath and the sound becomes erratic. Before you feel that the breath is almost finished, stop the sound, close your eyes and mouth, and bring your head forward to a comfortable position. Keeping the eyes closed and face relaxed, take one complete normal breath. Then, inhaling, open your eyes, roll them upward as you tilt your head, extend your tongue and continue. Repeat up to ten times.

## PRACTICE 7

# Neti

SOME OF MY EARLY and most unpleasant childhood memories are of being recurrently treated at a public hospital for nasal polyps and chronic sinusitis. I won't go into the gory details except to say that they are (literally) burned into the memory. I suffered from almost continuous sinus infections and the accompanying devastating headaches until I was twenty-two, when I was introduced to the practice of Neti. For the last thirty-two years, I have been totally free of this condition.

In this practice, warm saline water is allowed to flow through the nasal passages, using a specially designed container. When practiced correctly, it is very gentle and comfortable, and not at all similar to getting water up your nose either at the beach or in a swimming pool.

The water is at body temperature and the salt concentration should be about the same as that of your blood. This is called an "isotonic" solution. If you've ever had a nosebleed, you will recall that you weren't aware of the blood until it actually left your nostrils. This was because the flowing blood had the same temperature and salt concentration as the blood in the thousands of tiny capillaries that line your nasal passage.

## Background and Benefits

The technique (the origins of which are lost) has a number of variations, all of which are designed to cleanse and either stimulate or soothe the upper respiratory tract. The approach used in these practices is the most simple and generally therapeutic.

The obvious effects are the removal of excess mucus and promotion of efficient drainage from the sinuses. There are, however, deeper and subtle areas of action. The bottom of the brain and the space into which the water flows are only thinly separated by the roof of the nasopharynx. Through this roof the brain extends incredibly sensitive nerve endings from its "primitive" survival center where the "fight or flight" mechanism resides. These nerve endings constitute the olfactory bulb, the organ of our sense of smell. The comforting flow of warm water transmits a soothing, reflex sensation into the brain itself, promoting relaxation.

In classical yoga, anatomy and physiology, your sense of smell is directly connected to an energy center physically located in the area of the perineum, or pelvic floor.

In observations reported by Ashley Montagu in his book *Touching, the Human Significance of the Skin,* stimulus to this perineal area immediately after birth is crucial to the respiratory health of most mammals. This is why, when the mother is licking the newborn animal, she spends most of her time stimulating this area with her tongue, not because it tastes especially good. Newborn animals who are deprived of this stimulus inevitably suffer from impaired respiratory function and have difficulty becoming mobile. In this book he also makes a suggestion that there is a possible connection between Caesarean section deliveries and SIDS (Sudden Infant Death Syndrome).

The entire upper part of the respiratory tract is lined with a film of mucus which is always being propelled up and outward by millions of tiny hair-like structures called *cilia.* Neti stimulates this process also and can assist in ailments of this area such as bronchitis.

It can also be of great benefit in relieving headaches, promoting the best conditions for healing some diseases of the ears and throat, and also soothing the trigeminal nerve endings around the eyes. It is one of the most important natural treatments for epilepsy. In my stress management consultancy, I have also used it, with great success, to treat depression and hyperactivity.

Prepare your solution. Begin with approximately one level teaspoon of salt to half a liter (500 ml) or warm water, and then adjust the concentration to your comfort. Make sure it is around blood temperature.

Bend your head forward and turn it to the left, making sure that your mouth is open. Breathe through the mouth during the entire procedure. Introduce the nozzle of the container gently into the left nostril, so that the flared end forms a seal.

The water should flow easily into the nasopharynx (the cave behind the nasal opening) and then out through the opposite nostril. If the water tends more to run down the throat, adjust either or both the angle of the head and the angle of the pot. Repeat the process from the right side.

Sometimes there is a minor blockage to the flow. This can often be cleared by closing the other nostril with the finger and gently sucking the water through the blocked nostril, and spitting it out through the mouth. Once the blockage is cleared, proceed as normal.

If you don't happen to have access to one of the special pots (they are usually available through established yoga centers) you

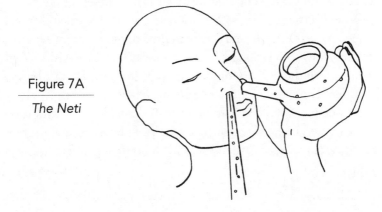

Figure 7A

*The Neti*

may like to try a small teapot. Be careful that the end of the spout is smooth and will not damage or irritate the nostrils. Alternatively, much of the cleansing effect of Neti, if not most of the soothing, can be obtained by using a bowl. Dip the nostril in, while closing the other one with the finger, and suck the water into the mouth. You should proceed with this method slowly and gently to avoid inhaling the water. I used this method for ten years before I was introduced to the special pots.

### Advanced Practice

Take water in through the mouth and, bending forward and down, expel the water through your nostrils. This level of practice may take some time to master. There are other more advanced practices, but they are not appropriate to describe here.

### Drainage

Immediately after practicing Neti, and especially if you are using the bowl method, it is crucial to drain any residual water from the area. This is done by bending forward from the waist so that the head is hanging downward and exhaling rapidly several times through both nostrils. You can clear what may sometimes be copious amounts of mucus by closing one nostril and gently blowing through the open one. I say gently with some emphasis as, if you blow forcefully, it is possible to force residual water into the opening of the eustachian tube which leads to the ear. Raise and lower your head several times while continuing to bend forward at the waist and repeat the process.

When we were living in New Orleans, where I learned this technique, my wife Angela and I were invited to dinner at an expensive restaurant by some friends. I finished my afternoon "Airlock" procedures with the practice of Neti, but was in too much of a hurry to get dressed and leave for the restaurant to bother with the drainage.

At one point, I stood leaning over the shoulder of our hostess to discuss a menu item. The haughty waiter was hovering and everyone was shocked to see what seemed an interminable stream of water pour from my left nostril onto the starched linen tablecloth. All ended well as the event provided a great conversation focus for the evening and provided me with an opportunity to expound on the value of the technique. Don't forget to drain, as the consequences may not only be inconvenient, they may be embarrassing.

# PRACTICE 8

# Nauli

IN 1979, I WAS approached by one of my students after an Integral Yoga class at my center in Perth, Western Australia. He was a man in his mid-fifties, and had been studying with me for a little more than a year. He asked if there were any specific yoga practices for the relief or cure of hiatus hernia, from which he had suffered for a couple years. I immediately responded that there was indeed something he could do to at least help the symptoms.

I proceeded to instruct him in Nauli. He was sufficiently fit, and had adequate muscular control to perform this, albeit without a great deal of definition at first attempt. I gave very specific, graduated instructions for him to apply over a three-month period, and asked him to keep me informed of his progress.

After he had left the center that evening, I thought I had better check in some of my reference books. On turning to Nauli, I was disappointed to read: "This practice is to be avoided by sufferers of hernia." After my initial reaction (which can best be described as "Ooops!"), I deliberated whether to call him and explain that I had found a prohibition for the instructions I had given him.

After some very ruthless self-examination, I concluded that my initial response to his request for help was intuitively correct and in fact, felt perfectly appropriate. The whole response to his question had been spontaneous; I had made no mental reference to any information on the condition whatsoever. It had been a self-to-self connection. I decided to wait and see what time would bring.

Three weeks passed without appropriate opportunity to monitor his progress, until, after his regular class, he asked to see me. After four days of practice, his symptoms had disappeared completely. He said, "I didn't want to report to you until I was sure it was permanent and now I am. Thank you." He remained symptom-free for the remainder of the year and subsequently reported that his general vitality was greatly improved and that his digestion was "superb."

It wasn't until 1989, in Hobart, Tasmania, that I had occasion to analyze the mechanics of the application of Nauli to this condition. A seventy-one year-old woman, grossly overweight, with emphysema, arthritis and a number of other conditions, asked me if there was anything yoga could do for hiatus hernia.

The hiatus hernia had only recently been diagnosed and although she was a little relieved that a name had been given for a condition that wasn't life threatening, she was still experiencing much distress.

She was obviously no candidate for Nauli. I answered in my habitual affirmative and said that there was something she could do herself. I very quickly analyzed the 1979 case. It was like looking at a three-dimensional color representation of the process taking place. I saw that when the abdominal rectus muscles were isolated and pushed forward, this created a partial vacuum that allowed the constricted part of the stomach to be released.

I asked her to wait until morning, when her stomach would be empty, and to drink as much lukewarm water as she could manage (at least 1.5 liters) and to drink it very quickly. After drinking the water as fast as she could, I asked her to rise up on her toes, stretching her arms above her head—then suddenly to drop her weight back down on to her heels.

Next morning she followed the instructions exactly, bumping down with her heels several times in succession. She felt (in her words) "something give inside." From that time she remained completely symptom-free until 1992, at which time I lost contact with her.

## Background and Benefits

The technique consists of consciously isolating the large columnar muscles at the front of your abdomen and then rotating them, self-massaging all the organs in your abdominal cavity. The quality and depth of this massage cannot be duplicated by any external method.

The liver, pancreas, spleen, whole lower digestive tract, reproductive organs, kidneys and bladder are all toned and residual unwanted accumulations milked out, disposed of by your blood and lymphatic system. The overall effect is to dramatically raise your level of vitality and energy.

Do this in front of a mirror. Make sure that your stomach is empty. Stand with your feet slightly more than shoulder-width apart. Bend your knees slightly and, keeping your back straight, bend forward from your waist so that your hands can be placed palms downward at your knees, while keeping your elbows locked and arms straight.

**Phase One:** Exhale completely and forcefully through your mouth, lower your chin into the hollow at the base of your throat and keep your lungs empty. With a moderate downward pressure on your thighs to assist you, draw your belly back towards your spine. Hold for one second only, let the contraction suddenly relax, releasing the pressure in your arms, and then apply the contraction again immediately.

Repeat this process as many times as you can comfortably manage while keeping your lungs empty. Always stay within the limitations of your comfortable breath capacity, very gradually increasing the number of contractions you can perform during one external breath retention. At first there may not be much discernible movement of your abdomen, but with regular daily practice, you will eventually be able to proceed to the next phase.

**Note:** When you reach the limit of your breath capacity and before you breathe in again, first always try to exhale a little more. This opens the airway and avoids a sudden, uncontrolled inrush of air.

**Phase Two:** When you are capable of performing around twenty contractions in the one breath, you will be ready to move to this phase. In classical yoga terminology it is called *Uddiyana Bandha*.

Proceed as for phase one, but, when you have drawn your belly back towards your spine, raise your shoulders and your ribcage and try to lift your abdomen up towards your chest cavity. Hold this contraction for as long as comfortable. When you are ready to release, lower your shoulders, relax your ribcage, then relax your belly, remembering to breathe out a little before you inhale.

By the time you become proficient at Phase Two, you will already be experiencing considerable benefits from the practice. Many digestive disorders are rectified, even at this stage of the practice. It is also especially applicable to people suffering from diabetes because of the stimulus to your pancreas.

**Phase Three:** Proceed as for Phase Two, applying a strong and comprehensive abdominal contraction. Bear down, applying pressure with your arms to your thighs and push your two large muscle columns forward, isolating them ventrally. The feeling is rather like trying to push your navel outward while keeping your abdomen sucked in.

Hold for a few seconds then draw everything in and upward in the Uddiyana Bandha. Repeat as many times as you can while comfortably keeping your breath out. Concentrate on achieving high quality muscular definition, rather than quantity of isolations. When the definition is good, you are ready to proceed to Phase Four.

**Phase Four:** In this stage, you are trying to separately isolate your two sides. Proceed as for Phase Two, applying the contraction. Bear down on your right side only, leaving your left side as relaxed as you can. The left side of your abdomen should be concave, while your right muscular column is pushed forward.

Relax the pressure on your right side, drawing everything again up into the Uddiyana Bandha. Repeat the process on your left side. You will probably find that the definition is better on one side than the other. If this is so, work on the weaker side until it equals the stronger. Again, concentrate on quality rather than the number of repetitions.

**Phase Five:** In this final stage, the aim is applying isolations alternately, creating a churning action. The Uddiyana Bandha needs to be quite strong as, while you are transferring the emphasis from one side to the other, it is responsible for the inner churning action. It takes time to develop the knack of moving with control from one isolation to the other to produce the deep massaging effect.

Isolate your left side, then slowly relax it, drawing it, with control, back towards your spine. When it is almost retracted, relinquish the pressure of your left arm and transfer it to your right, pushing your right muscular column outward. Just as you reach maximum isolation of your right side, start bearing down on your left and reduce the pressure being applied on the right. By the time your left side is at maximum isolation, your right side will be relaxed and concave again.

Work at perfecting the movement slowly, developing total control of each phase of the circular motion. Change the direction of your rotation from time to time, but always finish the session with a clockwise movement (if you were observing the circle being described by looking down at it from above) as this assists the natural peristaltic action in your large intestine.

Once the technique has been mastered, it can be used at various times throughout your day, even while seated in front of your computer. It also is a base practice for advanced internal cleansing procedures, but these require personal instruction.

You will feel its effects not simply on the physiological level; you are also very likely to experience a dramatic increase in assertiveness and general self-confidence.

# PRACTICE 9

# The Relaxation Pose

THIS IS THE BEST physical position in which to experience true relaxation. In simple terms, it involves lying on your back. First of all, it creates a situation where your heart no longer has to pump uphill to the brain, or maintain adequate pressure to ensure the return of venous blood from the legs. Your blood pressure is quickly reduced (normalized).

## The Practice

Lying on your back on a comfortable level surface, separate your feet to about shoulder width and allow them to fall outwards. Turn the palms of your hands upward so that the backs of your hands are in contact with the floor. This is important, as your fingers are richly supplied with nerves and pressure receptors that constantly relay information to your brain. When your hands are turned upward, this flow of information, or stimulus, is suspended. For you to be comfortable, it may mean that your arms have to be a considerable distance out from your sides. Experiment with this until it feels right.

More often with men, especially when they have considerable development of their upper arms, and if the practice is done for extended periods, it may be advisable to support the backs of the hands with small cushions or folded towels, so that the elbows are slightly bent. This prevents discomfort in your elbow joints.

Check that your head and body are in a straight line. It is advisable, especially for extended practice, to place a small sponge at the back of your skull, as pressure here can become a distraction. Close your eyes.

Having assumed the basic position, you are now ready to briefly explore its benefits or proceed further and deeper into the practice of Conscious Relaxation. If you only have five or ten minutes to spare and you want the maximum benefit, the swiftest pathway to relaxation is awareness of your breath.

However, before entering into breath awareness, mentally journey to all the points of contact of your body with the floor and briefly feel the exact contact point of each part in this sequence: heels, calves, backs of your thighs, buttocks, lower back, middle back, upper back, shoulder blades, backs of your hands, elbows, shoulders, and back of your head.

Bring your awareness now to the flow of air in your nostrils. The purpose here is not to regulate, but rather to relinquish all control over your breathing while becoming increasingly sensitive to, and aware of, the effortless movement of the air in and out of your nostrils. Cooler air enters your nose with inhalation, and warmer air leaves with exhalation.

As you inhale easily, mentally repeat, "I know I'm breathing in," and, as you exhale, "I know I'm breathing out." Try not to let a single breath slip past without you being aware of every millimeter of its journey in your nostrils. Once you're fully aware, count each breath backwards to zero.

The number at which you choose to start is limited only by the time you have to spend in the pose. When you begin, you will probably breathe at around six to eight breaths per minute. As you move deeper into the practice, and relaxation settles in, the rate will drop automatically, sometimes to as low as two breaths per minute. Thirty breaths is certainly enough to begin to feel the difference, and will probably take about five minutes.

Note: It is important to make absolutely sure that you will not be disturbed during practice, so lock the door, communicate your intent to staff or family, and switch off the telephone. It is also important that you avoid all physical movement once you have adjusted your position, until you finish the process.

In the early stages of your practice, you may often be distracted by itches that really have no identifiable source. Rather than becoming agitated by these and wishing they were not there, try to just let them be, and go on with the practice. They will often simply fade away. If they become unbearable and you really have to scratch, then try to make the movement slowly, with awareness and sensitivity, disturbing yourself as little as possible.

The Relaxation Pose can swiftly restore balance to both circulatory and nervous systems, as well as being mentally refreshing. It establishes the physical and chemical inner climate for the practice of Conscious Relaxation.

## CONSCIOUS RELAXATION

A more comprehensive description of this technique and its benefits is given in Chapter 5, "An Antidote for Stress." (You may wish to record the following instructions on audiotape, to play back when you begin practicing.)

### The Practice

Having established the Relaxation Pose up to the point of being aware of the contact points of your body with the floor, proceed as follows:

Move your awareness and sensitivity very swiftly around the whole body several times, just like a spark jumping from point to point, following the sequence from your heels to the back of your head.

Feel the gentle contact of the lids of your closed eyes and develop the feeling that your eyes are falling back, totally relaxed in their sockets. Feel the contact of your lips gently touching, and the muscles of your cheeks and jaw totally relaxed.

Now become aware of your body as a complete unit. Mentally repeat and feel, "Whole body, whole body," leaving nothing out. Think of your body as one homogeneous unit. Feel your entire body all at the same instant, and mentally repeat, "Whole body."

Tell yourself, "I am practicing Conscious Relaxation and I am awake. I am awake." The purpose is not to sleep but to remain aware and conscious throughout. Now and then you will have to check up on yourself as the relaxation proceeds, and be sure that you are awake. As relaxation deepens, it is natural for sleep to come, but don't let yourself go into it. Remain awake and aware.

## Resolution

It is at this point that you can repeat your resolve, if you have clearly formulated one. It should be positive and repeated three times with the conviction that it will come to fruition.

## Sound Awareness

Become aware of external sound. Welcome every sound as it comes. Don't try to distinguish in terms of pleasant or unpleasant, but create a welcome attitude toward every sound, no matter what it might be. Keep your awareness moving from sound to sound. As soon as you are aware of a particular sound, immediately seek out the next one. Go from loud to soft. The external sounds: traffic, sounds in the distance, outside the building and those inside. The internal sounds: the subtle sounds of your own breathing, heart beating. Continue to enter deeply into the faculty of hearing. There is nowhere to go and nothing to do at this point but to listen, and to listen totally.

The intensity of this experience should be as if all your other senses were unavailable to you and, without generating any tension, as if your very life depended on being able to detect every tiny sound. From time to time, try to become aware of the sound between sounds, the underlying substratum from which all these sounds proceed and into which they all eventually subside. Continue.

## Breath Awareness

Now become aware of the ocean of air that surrounds you, stretching away infinitely on all sides, the ocean of air in which we live as a fish lives in water. Become aware of its vastness. Relinquish all control over your breathing process. Let it happen effortlessly. As inhalation proceeds, you simply offer no obstruction, no impediment to the inflow of the ocean of air, allowing it to permeate your entire body and, with exhalation, create the experience of simply letting go.

Become aware of this flow exclusively in your nostrils, its twin streams of air entering your nostrils and moving upwards into your head. Cooler air entering with the inhalation and warmer air leaving with the exhalation. Continue moving your awareness closer and closer to this flow in your nostrils. Twin streams entering, moving upward into your head, and at a certain point they seem to meet, to merge. Be aware of this meeting point. As you exhale, it is from this point that the twin streams diverge, separate and move down and out.

Now begin your backward counting from 21 to zero. "I know I'm breathing in. I know I'm breathing out—21. I know I'm breathing in. I know I'm breathing out—20," and so on, back to zero. Treat each breath as a separate and unique opportunity for increasing your sensitivity to the movement of the air in your nasal passage. Don't let the process become mechanical but continue to intensify your exploration of each breath.

As you move down through the low numbers toward zero, it's possible you may drift off to sleep as you enter into the borderline state. Be alert, remain awake and aware. When you resist the urge to drift, and can enter fully into this sleepless "sleep," you will feel a great change as you go into a deeper level of awareness. Start your counting now. Continue.

## Journey Through Your Body

Let your breath awareness just fall away. We're going on a journey through all the body, through the parts of your body. Move your awareness to each part as its name is called; try to have a quick mental picture of the part concerned. It's as if you are exploring with hundreds of tiny mental fingers, feeling the whole part, not just the external form, but the entire area.

Bring your awareness to the thumb of your right hand. We will move quite quickly—try to maintain your contact with the flow of instructions. It is most important that you do not fall off to sleep. Tell yourself now, "I am aware. I am awake."

The thumb of your right hand, index finger, middle finger, fourth finger, little finger, palm, back of your hand, wrist, forearm, elbow, upper arm, shoulder, armpit, side, slide your awareness down the right side over your ribcage to your waist. The bony projection of your right hip, groin, large muscles of your right thigh, upper and lower, your knee, back of the knee, inside of the knee, kneecap, calf muscle, shin, ankle joint, upper surface of your foot, heel, sole of your foot, big toe, second toe, third toe, fourth toe, little toe.

Come straight away to your left side, to your left hand and the thumb of your left hand. The thumb of your left hand, index finger, middle finger, fourth finger, little finger, palm, back of your hand, wrist, forearm, elbow, upper arm, shoulder, armpit, side, slide your awareness down the left side over your ribcage to your waist.

The bony projection of your left hip, groin, large muscles of your left thigh, upper and lower, your knee, back of your knee, inside of your knee, kneecap, calf muscle, shin, ankle joint, upper surface of your foot, heel, sole of your foot, big toe, second toe, third toe, fourth toe, little toe.

Whole left leg, whole left leg. Mentally repeat "Whole left leg" and try to feel it from the tips of your toes to your hip joint, all at the same time. "Whole left leg."

Whole right leg, whole right leg. Mentally repeat "Whole right leg" and try to feel it from the tips of your toes to your hip joint, all at the same time. "Whole right leg."

Left buttock, right buttock, sacrum (the triangular-shaped bone at the base of your spinal column), lower back, left side of your back, right side of your back, left shoulder blade, right shoulder blade, whole spinal column, whole spinal column.

Whole left arm. From the tips of your fingers to your shoulder, at a glance, try to feel it all at the same moment. "Whole left arm."

Whole right arm. From the tips of your fingers to your shoulder, at a glance, try to feel it all at the same moment with one swift movement of your mind. "Whole right arm."

Back of your neck, back of your head, top of your head, left side of your head, right side of your head, forehead, mid-eyebrow point, left eye, relax your eye in the socket, and your eyelid, right eye, and your eyelid, left nostril, right nostril, nose tip, upper lip, lower lip, left cheek, right cheek, chin, jawline from ear to ear, throat, hollow at the base of your throat, left side of your chest, right side of your chest, your breastbone, upper abdomen between your breastbone and your navel, the navel itself, lower abdomen between your navel and your pubic bone, pubic bone, left groin, genitals, right groin, pubic bone, navel, center of your breastbone, hollow at the base of your throat, mid-eyebrow point.

Be aware of your whole body, whole body as one unit. Try to feel whole body at once and mentally repeat "Whole body." Become aware of your breathing once again, but in a particular way. Try to feel that you are breathing, not just with your lungs, but rather that, as you inhale, the breath is entering your body through every pore, over your whole skin surface.

As you inhale, your breath effortlessly enters your body over your whole skin. Create for yourself the feeling of expansion and lightness within your body. As you exhale, there's no sense of contraction, but rather, just letting go—an inner relaxation. Continue to create for yourself the feeling of expansion and lightness with inhalation and then the feeling of letting go, inner relaxation, with exhalation. Continue.

Try to feel that your whole body is becoming so light that, if a breeze came, your body would drift just like a balloon on a string. Feel that it is becoming so large that it fills the entire room. You can create this feeling for yourself. Go on deepening your awareness in this way.

Please shift the emphasis, shift the focus of your breath awareness, to the exhalation. I want you to feel that you are breathing out through the very center of your breastbone, as if there were a tube or a passage that extends from the center of your breastbone back down through your chest cavity towards your spinal cord. The breathing is taking place in this imaginary passageway and, with each exhalation, I want you to create the feeling of totally and utterly letting go. With each exhalation, letting go more and more.

Let go of anger, let go of expectation, fear, let go of all tension and link the letting go with this outward breath, through your heart center. Continue.

Hold onto nothing, totally and utterly letting go. Let go of sadness also, or disappointment. Totally letting go. Surrendering the inner space, within your heart, within your chest, to the external space—just let go. Continue.

Once again, become aware of your whole body where it is in contact with the floor. Be aware of the dimensions of your body, be aware of its weight, its solidity and mentally repeat again, "Whole body—whole body" and try to feel it.

Mentally repeat, "Now the practice is finished." Be aware of external sounds and all sensory information. Consciously externalize your awareness. Keep your eyes closed, but now you can begin to release the position. Move with awareness, move with sensitivity, gradually releasing the position. Move your fingers and your toes, then have a good stretch, turn from side to side and finally, still keeping your eyes closed, sit up.

Open your eyes very gradually, slowly, and carry the feeling with you throughout the rest of your day.

# PRACTICE 10

## Inner Silence

HOW MANY TIMES HAS a random thought come to mind and sucked you down a corridor of painful memory or speculation, changing your experience of whatever you were engaged in at the time?

To understand someone or something, you have to spend time studying, observing, and becoming familiar with their expression and characteristics. Our mind itself, with its undeniable power to determine the course of our lives, rarely becomes the subject of this intimate study. We think, or thoughts come, and we do our best to deal with the sunshine or storms they create.

This practice is a structured and systematic way of developing insight and friendliness towards your mind, and also a way of liberating yourself from its power to negatively influence your perceptions and responses by understanding the way it works. There are five defined stages and we will go through them in turn. (Suggestion: You may wish to record the following instructions on audiotape, to play back when you begin practicing.)

### Stage One
Assume the Relaxation Pose. It can be performed sitting in any easy position, as long as your spine is comfortably erect and you can

remain still. Gently close your eyes and keep them closed. Make any small adjustments to your position necessary for your comfort and then, from this point on, do not move.

In this first stage, create an attitude of impartial witness to all information coming to you through your senses. Develop this observer faculty so that, later in the practice, you will be able to witness the activity of your mind. Begin with your sense of hearing.

Become aware of all the sounds coming to you through your ears. To crystallize this witness, apply your awareness to the experience of hearing by analyzing its components. The first is the sound itself. Next, the medium of perception—in this case, your ears. The third component is you who are registering the sound coming to you through your ears. So as you listen, the form of the awareness becomes more conscious, "the sound, my ears, I, who am listening." Continue deepening your awareness of hearing; seek out all levels of sound, all the while maintaining the consciousness that "I am hearing the sound."

As you move through your senses, it is important to maintain the knowledge that you are consciously interacting with them, and also to establish a welcoming attitude to each sensation. Don't differentiate between a pleasant and unpleasant stimulus. Welcome every sound, no matter what it might be. Continue.

Now become aware of the messages coming through your sense of touch. Feel all the points of body contact with the floor. Feel where your clothing contacts your body, where the air touches the skin surface of your face and hands. You experience sensations in the physical body, through your sense of touch, and don't become disturbed or distracted by these, but rather stay conscious of experiencing them.

All these messages, through the senses of hearing, touch, taste, smell and sight, constantly flow below the level of your conscious awareness each and every day. Now you deliberately engage your awareness in the processes, with the feeling "I am the witness. I am the observer of these sensations." Register any and all touch sensations and know that you are being aware of them.

Now bring your awareness to the tongue. As if you are exploring with hundreds of tiny mental fingers along the upper surface, from the tip of the tongue towards the back of the mouth and along both edges. Focus on any experience of taste that you can detect: salty, sweet or bitter. Be aware "I am tasting this." Continue.

From your tongue, move into the area of the nose. High in the roof of the cave inside your head, behind the nostrils, is a tiny area of sensitivity. This is your organ of smell. Try to locate this point and become aware of the flow of the air exclusively in this area. Detect any perfume, odor or scent, even the slightest residual smell, and be aware that you are experiencing it. Continue.

Come to the space in front of your closed eyes and be aware of whatever you can see there. It may be colors or shapes, vague forms, or it may simply be warm darkness. Be aware of the act of seeing: "Visual field—my eyes—I who am seeing." Continue.

This completes Stage One. The progressive introversion of the sense awareness brings a feeling of calm and tranquillity. You can use this process at any time throughout your day: riding on a bus, waiting for an appointment, whenever there are a few moments to spare. There will always be distractions and disturbances, but as you go on developing the attitude of a dispassionate witness, an observer, while engaged in any activity, you begin to crystallize your sense of "self" and become more and more centered.

## Stage Two

Now you move from physical awareness to awareness of the thinking process. Become aware of your thoughts as they come and go.

Here you should not attempt to control your thoughts in any way. Only resolve to remain awake and aware of each thought as it surfaces. Give yourself total freedom in this stage to allow any thought at all to come. Be alert to the arrival of any thought, whatever its content. Some thought processes are predominantly visual, and some almost exclusively verbal. It really doesn't matter what yours may be, as long as you create the feeling of being a witness to them.

Sometimes, even in the early stages of practice, unpleasant or painful thoughts may come. If and when they do, it is because they need to, and you need to let them. Presumably, the fact that you feel and interpret the thought as unpleasant or painful means that you would rather not be affected by it, so these thoughts are like splinters in your well-being. To extract a splinter, the first thing you have to do is look at it.

Tell yourself, "This is not going on now. Now I have just allowed this thought to come so that I can observe it." The secret of dispelling the power of a thought to affect us negatively is, simply, to observe it. Study it. Be aware, "I am watching this thought."

When you assert this witnessing faculty, the link of expected intimacy between the thought and your capacity to be disturbed or distressed by it is dissolved. You have put a little gap between you and that thought and it becomes less possible for it to suck you into some unchosen area of grief, or anger, or depression. If a powerfully painful experience comes, observe—witness. Remember "This experience is not going on now. Now I am watching this thought. I am the witness."

After some time of watching the thoughts but not being swept away by them, you are ready to move into Stage Three, the stage of deliberately choosing a thought.

Remember, Stage One was the exploration of your senses: touch, hearing, taste, smell, and sight and the creation of your witnessing. Stage Two was the turning inward of your observation towards the thoughts themselves—witnessing, but with no control. Now comes choice. Now comes control.

## Stage Three

Choose a thought for yourself. Do not allow any spontaneous thought to intervene. Whether you choose some mundane, unimportant thought, or something of great intensity, it is your choice. If you are aware of something near the surface that you need to deal with, then do it. But do it only according to your preference, your courage, and according to how well you are able to enter and sustain the witnessing faculty.

Choose any thought. Maintain it. Observe it. Allow it to grow and develop its associations, but don't allow any unconnected thought to intrude. Keep to the theme of the original thought you have chosen. Be aware "I have chosen this thought and I am observing it." Continue.

After some time of watching this chosen thought, you now develop the faculty of being able to discard a thought at will. When you are ready, dispose of that chosen thought with a swift decisive act of will. If it is verbal, cut off the words and, if it is visual, dissolve the picture. Continue.

Now immediately hold yourself in readiness, be alert. Choose another, totally different thought and go on in the same way—witnessing—observing, not getting sucked in by the thought but preserving the gap, "I am doing the practice. I have chosen the thought so that I can observe it." Choose several separate thoughts and deal with them in this way. Continue.

Again, with a sudden and decisive movement of the mind and the will, let that thought go. Let it dissolve. Hold yourself in readiness for the next level.

### Stage Four

Just as you allowed spontaneous thoughts to come in the second stage, you allow them now. But with the great difference that, in this stage of practice, after permitting the spontaneous thought to come, you only allow it to remain for a short period.

When you are ready, you consciously dispose of it, suddenly and decisively and then hold yourself in readiness, as a witness, waiting for another spontaneous thought to surface. Take your time. Entertain the thought only as long as you choose, then discard it. Continue.

Remember, "I am doing the Practice. I am watching the thought." Let the thoughts come of their own accord, but you decide their moments of departure. Good or bad, agitated or pleasant thoughts; don't discriminate. Don't be thrown. Stay alert. Be a witness. Let several thoughts come spontaneously and practice disposing of them in turn. Go on with this practice.

In the next and final stage, the aim is to prevent a single thought from fully forming. Use the skill developed in the third and fourth stages—the ability to dissolve a thought at will.

## Stage Five

Here you become a warrior, a sentry of your mind. Don't let a single thought form. In the instant you become aware that a thought has arrived, dispose of it. Hold yourself in readiness, alert for the next one. And go on dissolving the pictures, cutting off the words. The only thought in the mind during this period is "I will have no thought."

Sometimes the onrush of thought is swift, and at other times, there are spaces. When one thought has gone and another not yet arrived, this space is the gateway to the deepest realms of Inner Silence. If it presents itself, unmistakably, enter it with simply the awareness "I am." Within this space, this gap in the process of thinking, also lies deep restoration of mental energy.

Continue, be alert and aware. This is not suppression according to any preference or fear. You don't care if a thought is wonderfully positive and wholesome or disturbingly intense. Here, in this final stage, all of them are dispatched before they can fully surface. Stay alert. Be a sentry, "I will have no thought."

Be aware also of the space between the thoughts, the space in your head into which the thoughts come, and into which they are dissolved. Continue.

Now the practice is over. Externalize your awareness. Hear the sounds. Feel your body sensations. Become aware of the weight of your body pressing on the floor. The practice is over, but it doesn't end here. Take this developing awareness, the witnessing faculty, and awaken it regularly throughout your day.

The essence of the practice is to use it in the midst of activity: while you are working, traveling, relating, or resting. Develop a friendly relationship with your mind. Get to know it. Use it, rather than be at its mercy. Even if you only dip into the awareness for a few moments, in those moments there is no stress.

Every now and then, activate the witness. Ask yourself, "What am I thinking now? What am I thinking now?" At any time of day or night, develop the habit of coming back to square one: placing yourself in the present moment, and become aware of the play of the mind.

Slowly begin to release the position of your body, moving your fingers and toes with the awareness, "I am moving the fingers. I am moving my toes." Awaken the whole body and bring it back into movement, into activity. Have a good stretch, turn from side to side and finally sit up. Open your eyes and go on with awareness.

## The Potential of Inner Silence

The various stages of this technique provide the basis for other methods and applications, either abbreviated and integrated into the daily life, or deepened and explored for purposes of mental and emotional health, and for accessing creative potential.

**Body Check:** You can apply the process of becoming aware of sensory information used in Stage One at any time. It is better, if you plan to incorporate it into your routine, to establish regular moments or intervals, according to your schedule. In this way it is easier to develop the habit of using the tool.

**Relaxing the Mind:** When the witnessing faculty is applied to the thinking process by stopping at any time, by becoming present and asking yourself, "What am I thinking now?"—then there is an automatic and swift mental relaxation. This is established as the awareness is introverted and the power connection with any unproductive thought is severed. You are no longer at its mercy.

**Liberation from Repetitive, Obsessive Thoughts:** The capacity to suddenly dispose of thoughts at will, which you progressively developed in Stages Three and Four, is invaluable when you are plagued by worries and anxieties. This is especially useful when it is not at all appropriate to consider whatever the source of the problem may be. You acknowledge the thought, or the theme, and tell yourself "I'll get to this later; right now I'm busy," and with a mental flick of the wrist, you dispose of it.

**Critical Incident Defusing:** Occasionally, there will be major, well-defined stress incidents in our lives. The faster we can deal with these in terms of their mental and emotional impact, the sooner we can get on with living, unimpaired by grief, regret, fear, or anger. The substance of Stage Three, wherein you choose a thought for yourself to observe, then later dispose of it at will, is a platform from which you can swiftly and comprehensively clear these experiences.

**Associative Defusing:** Where there is anxiety or fear of certain situations or possible events, the elements of Stage Three can be used in a process of creative visualization. Mentally create a situation, paying great attention to detail, in which you feel and perform in a calm, secure, happy, and powerful way. Then bring in aspects of those situations that usually cause anxiety or fear and see yourself dealing with them easily and capably. The ripples will spread into your external life, and you will cease to be disturbed by these events and, specifically, you will cease to be disturbed by their anticipation. This is the art of using your mind—not being dominated by it.

# PRACTICE 11

# Sun Salutation

THIS IS A COMPREHENSIVE form of potentially aerobic exercise that positively affects not only your major muscles, joints and spinal column, but also your internal organs. It requires no special equipment and, for best results, should be performed in the early morning after bathing, although it may be used anytime to restore flagging energy and mental vitality.

When you use it regularly, it is best to gradually and progressively increase the number of rounds you perform daily. Starting with no more than three rounds, add a round per week until you reach the number required for your own fitness maintenance schedule. Depending on your other activities during the day, this should be between twelve to twenty rounds per day.

This gradual approach is important, not only to safely increase the levels of work on your skeletal, muscular, and cardiovascular systems, but also in terms of making the accompanying process of toxin elimination more comfortable. The Sun Salutation does not simply work on these bodily systems, but also encourages the removal and subsequent elimination through the skin, lungs, digestive, and urinary systems of waste that may have accumulated in tissue and organs as a result of inappropriate diet, lifestyle, and undischarged stress.

It consists of a flowing movement, synchronized with your breath, through a series of twelve positions. One complete round consists of two repetitions of the sequence.

**Position 1:** Stand for a few moments, feet together and palms of your hands gently touching your chest. Close your eyes and relax your whole body. Breathe normally for a while, then exhale fully.

**Position 2:** As you inhale, separate your palms, extend your arms out in front of you and, in time with the inhalation, raise them above your head. At the top of the movement and breath, your head and upper back are inclined slightly backward.

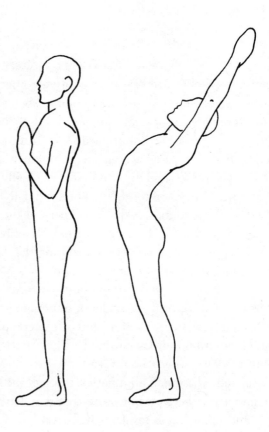

Practice 11A–B

*Sun Salutation
Position 1 (left)*

*Sun Salutation
Position 2 (right)*

**Position 3:** Slowly exhale and, keeping your arms extended, bend forward from your waist until, at the end of the exhalation, your hands are as close as comfortable to the floor while keeping your legs straight.

**Position 4:** As you inhale, while bending your right knee, lower your pelvis and stretch your left leg back, toes and knee in contact with the floor. At the same time your head is inclined backward, spine extended and gaze directed at the ceiling. Your weight is supported on your hands, right foot, and left knee and toes.

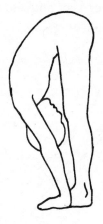

Practice 11C

*Sun Salutation*
*Position 3*

Practice 11D

*Sun Salutation*
*Position 4*

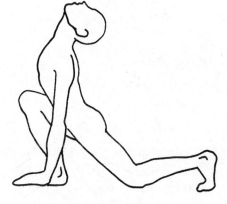

**Position 5:** Supporting your weight mainly on your hands and right foot, exhale while raising your buttocks in the air, straightening and extending your left leg back so that your foot comes to rest alongside the right. Allow your head to hang. Your heels are as close to the floor as your straightened legs will permit. Having arrived at this position at the end of the exhalation, keep your breath outside for a few moments as you move into Position 6.

**Position 6:** Keeping your breath outside for a few moments, lower your body to the floor by bending your knees and elbows. Chin, chest, palms, knees, and toes are in contact with the floor, while your buttocks are kept raised so that the lower belly and pubic bone are suspended.

Practice 11E

*Sun Salutation
Position 5*

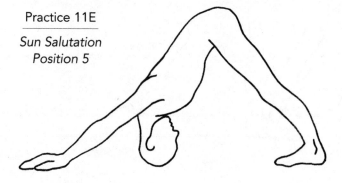

Practice 11F

*Sun Salutation
Position 6*

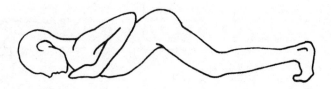

**Position 7:** Exhale just a little more, to open the airway, then, as you slowly inhale, raise your head and upper back, straightening your arms and making sure the pubic bone is in contact with the floor. Relax your lower back in this position.

**Position 8:** Exhale, straightening your arms and legs, while raising your buttocks again as you did in Position 5.

Practice 11G

*Sun Salutation*
*Position 7*

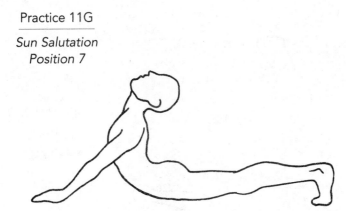

Practice 11H

*Sun Salutation*
*Position 8*

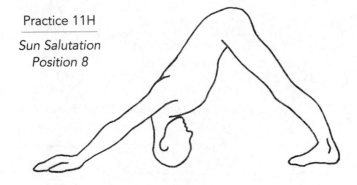

**Position 9:** Supporting your weight on your hands, left knee, and toes, slowly inhale as you bend your right knee, bringing your right foot in one fluid movement to rest between your hands. Arch the head and torso backward.

**Position 10:** Supporting your weight on your right leg and hands, exhale as you release your left leg and bring your left foot alongside the right foot. Straighten your legs and allow your hands to be as close to the floor as comfortable. This is the same as Position 3.

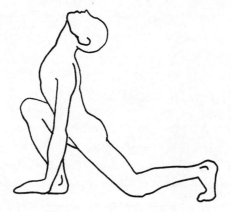

Practice 11I

*Sun Salutation
Position 9*

Practice 11J

*Sun Salutation
Position 10*

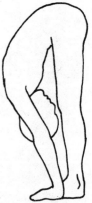

**Position 11:** As you slowly inhale, bring your extended arms, trunk, and head up to a repetition of Position 2. Lead the movement with your head, bringing your spine to the raised position vertebra by vertebra.

**Position 12:** Exhale as you come into this final position, which is exactly the same as Position 1.

This constitutes one half round. To complete a round, repeat the movements as above, except that in Position 4 your left leg is extended back, and in Position 9 your left foot is placed between your hands.

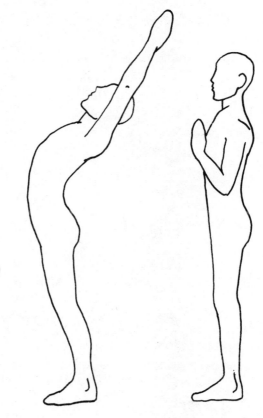

Practice 11K–L

*Sun Salutation
Position 11 (left)*

*Sun Salutation
Position 12 (right)*

# SUGGESTED READING

Airola, Paavo. *Are You Confused?: The Authoritative Answers to Controversial Questions*. Chicago: Health Plus Publications, 1971.

———. *How to Get Well: Dr. Airola's Handbook of Natural Healing*. Chicago: Health Plus Publications, 1984.

D'Adamo, Dr. Peter. *Eat Right For Your Type: The Individualized Diet Solution to Staying Healthy, Living Longer & Achieving Your Ideal Weight*. New York: Putnam Publishing Group, 1997.

Garrott, Geoffrey. *Ethics in Business: A Deeper Approach*. Hobart, Tasmania, Australia: Institute of Business Ethics, Inc., 1992.

Krishna, Gopi. *Kundalini: The Evolutionary Energy in Man*. Boston, MA: Shambhala Publications, 1971.

Meares, Dr. Ainslie. *Dialogue on Meditation, from the Quiet Place, a Kind of Believing*. Melbourne, Australia: Hill of Content, 1989.

Montagu, Ashley. *Touching: The Human Significance of the Skin*. New York: HarperCollins, 1986.

Motoyama, Dr. Hiroshi. *Theories of the Chakras: Bridge to Higher Consciousness*. Wheaton, IL: Theosophical Publishing House, 1989.

————. *Toward Superconsciousness: Meditational Theory and Practice*. Freemont, CA: Jain Publishing Co., 1990.

Mumford, Dr. Jonn. *Ecstasy Through Tantra*. St. Paul, MN: Llewellyn Publications, 1987.

Ornish, Dr. Dean. *Stress, Diet and Your Heart*. New York: New American Library, 1991.

Saraswati, Swami Satyananda. *Meditations from the Tantras*. Gosford, NSW, Australia: Satyananda Ashram, 1984.

Simonton, Carl, Stephanie Matthews, and James L. Creighton. *Getting Well Again*. New York: Bantam Books, 1992.

Toffler, Alvin. *Future Shock*. New York: Bantam Books, 1991.

Tompkins, Peter, and Christopher O. Bird. *The Secret Life of Plants*. New York: HarperCollins, 1989.

Watson, Lyall. *Supernature: A Natural History of the Supernatural*. London: Hodder and Stoughton, Ltd., 1973.

# Glossary

adrenaline: a stimulating hormone, or chemical trigger that affects muscles and circulation.

Airlock, The: the distinction you create between work and personal environments.

Autonomic Nervous System: the network of specialized cells which automatically controls body functions such as heart rate.

bioelectricity: the organized flow of energy that animates us; variously described in different traditions as Chi or Prana, demonstrated to exist empirically by Kirlian photography and the work of Dr. Hiroshi Motoyama.

Body Check: a quick method of centering by swiftly journeying with the awareness sequentially through the body; similar to Vipassana (Buddhist meditation technique) and based on the much older Tantric method of Nyasa.

Borderline state: also referred to as the hypnogogic state; just before sleep, when the flow of conscious sensory input has abated but consciousness is still present; Alpha state.

**Brain Massage:** a breathing technique for refreshing the brain and interrupting the flow of obsessive thought; based on Kapalabhati (Sanskrit: Skull Shining), one of the six central practices of Hatha Yoga.

**Camel Pose, The:** technique involving the large thigh muscles to adjust blood chemistry; ideal if your work is largely sedentary; based on Ushtrasana (Hatha Yoga Asana).

**carotid sinus receptors:** nerves in the throat directly connected to the part of the brain that monitors and adjusts such bodily functions as blood pressure.

**Centering Breath, The:** breathing technique that balances both energy and alternate brain hemisphere function; based on the Tantric practice of Anuloma Viloma (as distinct from the fifth Indian Pranayama of the same name).

**ch'i (or ki):** subtle, organized flow of energy (life force).

**Child Pose, The:** a technique for strengthening the immune system and addressing emotional imbalance; particularly useful in anxiety/depression; based on Shashankasana (Hatha Yoga Asana).

**cilia:** microscopically small hair-like structures that, by concerted movement, propel the lining film of mucus upwards in the upper respiratory tract.

**Conscious Relaxation:** a deeply restorative technique that can provide the equivalent of 4 hours sleep in 45 minutes; based on the method Yoga Nidra (evolved by Swami Satyananda), similar to autogenic training.

**diaphragm:** the sheet of muscle dividing the trunk into abdominal and thoracic cavities; it is the hardest working muscle in the body, being the prime mover in the breathing process.

**dream state:** one of the stages of sleep; REM state; essential for processing unresolved life events and amenable to preprogramming.

**habituation:** the process of getting so used to a level of stimulus that we cease to recognize it.

**Humming Bee, The:** breathing technique for swift access to relaxation; based on Bhramari Pranayama (Hatha Yoga), also one of the essential practices in Laya Yoga and Nada Yoga (Yoga of Sound).

**hypertension:** elevated blood pressure.

**Inner Silence:** conscious thinking technique for developing the witnessing faculty (Sanskrit: Sakshi Bhava: the attitude or feeling of being a knowing observer); based on the practice of Antar Mauna as developed by Swami Satyananda; particularly useful for releasing and defusing suppressed trauma and for debriefing after critical incidents.

**intercostal muscles:** the muscles between the ribs that promote expansion and contraction of the chest.

**Letting Go:** series of isolated muscular contractions, coordinated with the breath to discharge muscular tension.

**Maha Shakti:** the ocean of energy in which we live, just as a fish lives in water.

**Monitoring Breath, The:** subtle breathing technique for centering and maintaining equanimity; helps to regulate blood pressure (based on the Sanskrit: Ujjayi Pranayama).

**Nauli:** one of the six central practices of Hatha Yoga; progressively developing control of the large abdominal muscles so as to be able to give yourself a deep organic massage.

**Neti:** one of the six central practices of Hatha Yoga; irrigation of the nasal passages with warm salted water; removes accumulated airborne toxins and soothes the primitive brain.

**Non-Specific Tension (NST):** a maintained state of nervous tension that impairs judgment and function, for which no particular cause can be identified.

**Parasympathetic Nervous System:** the branch of the Autonomic Nervous System that is responsible for restoring balance after a crisis; the Relaxation Response.

**pineal:** a small, light-sensitive gland in the brain; previously believed to atrophy after puberty, especially in males, but now considered a partner of the pituitary gland in maintaining circadian rhythm. Regarded in Yoga Anatomy as the site of Ajna Chakra and the center of intuition.

**pituitary:** in the brain, sometimes called the master gland; orchestrates the entire chain of endocrine hormonal secretions, controlling growth and metabolism.

**prana:** life energy (ch'i) that flows along organized pathways and maintains mental and physical harmony.

**Relaxation Response:** see the Parasympathetic Nervous System; once thought to be an unconscious mechanism but now recognized as being accessible to conscious control.

**reticular activating system (RAS):** group of specialized cells at the top of the brainstem which controls generally unconscious functions such as temperature, heart rate, blood pressure, breathing.

**serotonin:** a compound in blood, a neurotransmitter; sometimes referred to as the relaxation hormone.

**Shaking All Over:** a system of swiftly increasing circulation to body joints in preparation for exercise.

**Six Events, The:** a painless way to reprogram yourself for centering by slipping the chosen technique (breath awareness, etc.) in alongside an already accepted part of your daily routine.

**Steady Gazing (Sanskrit: Trataka):** one of the six central practices of Hatha Yoga; a method of stabilizing concentration, centering and accessing memory by gazing at a fixed point.

**stress (chronic, acute):** a demand made upon your body and mind; chronic stress simply means that the experience has been going on for some time and acute stress is usually sudden.

**stress reaction:** activation of the Sympathetic Nervous System when your primitive brain identifies a situation as being threatening.

**Sun Salutation:** a system of exercising and energizing the body through a sequence of twelve consecutive positions.

**Sushumna (Sanskrit: nadi):** the central pathway in the Yogic energy body through which evolutionary energy, Kundalini, rises to illuminate the dormant areas of the brain; in the Staff of Aesculapius, it is represented by the central staff around the twin serpents (Ida Nadi: mental energy and Pingala Nadi: physical energy) are entwined around. It is recognized that Kundalini energy can only travel safely along this pathway (refer to the books of Gopi Krishna).

**thoracic cavity:** the upper section of the trunk; the chest, enclosing vital organs such as heart and lungs.

**Thunderbolt Pose, The (Sanskrit: Vajrasana):** the meditation pose of Zen Buddhism; ideal for maintaining spinal integrity and promoting excellent digestion.

**Tongue Lock, The (Sanskrit: Khechari Mudra):** placing the tip of the tongue against the hard or soft palate and exerting gentle pressure; a method of establishing and maintaining balanced brain hemisphere function. See Dr. Jonn Mumford's *Ecstasy Through Tantra.*

**tryptophane:** an essential dietary element; an amino acid.

**Uddiyana Bandha (Sanskrit):** a technique of Hatha Yoga; drawing the abdominal musculature back towards the spine and upward, compressing the abdominal contents.

**Unwinding:** preprogramming yourself for more efficient dreaming by going back through the day's events.

**Washroom Retreat, The:** a way to efficiently restore balance and center even in the busiest work environment by availing yourself for a few minutes in what may be the only private space.

yoga (Hatha): the science of establishing perfect harmony between mental and physical energies (the twin serpents twined around the Hermetic Staff); generally regarded as comprising postures (Sanskrit: asana) and breathing techniques (pranayama) but classically consisting of just six central practices called the Shatkarmas or Shatkriyas. Four of these are utilized in *Mastery of Stress:* Neti, Nauli, Kapalabhati and Trataka.

# INDEX

constipation, 15, 38, 82–83, 134, 160, 162

culture, Indian, xi, 125–126

circuit training, 54–55

deadlines, 97

defusing
fear, 64, 92–93, 134, 138, 184, 190, 192
anger, 31, 64, 76, 134, 146, 184, 188, 192
associative, 47, 192

depression, 44, 60, 134, 167, 188

diaphragm, 11, 66–67, 131

dreaming, 111, 114

duodenal ulcer, 81

electroencephalograph (EEG), 29–30, 145

electromagnetic fields, 86

endocrine system, 32

entertainment, 44, 162

epiglottis, 72, 102

ethics, 89–94

fear, 64, 92–93, 134, 138, 184, 190, 192

fight or flight syndrome, 9–11, 64, 110

fine motor control, 150

fire, 32, 35, 52, 141

fitness, 43, 54–56, 58, 161–162, 193

floor, 7, 10, 20, 36, 38–39, 57–59, 85, 102–104, 130, 133, 150–153, 162–163, 166, 177–179, 184, 186, 190, 195–198

food, 24, 28, 33–34, 43–44, 66, 72, 77–87, 114, 159

friendship, gift of, 106–107

gall bladder, 80

Garrott, Geoffrey, 89

gaseous exchange, 63

gastric ulcer, 80

gastro-colic reflex, 82

giving, 10, 92, 138

gout, 34

gravity, 39, 81, 131–133

gym, 54–55, 100, 123

habituation, 13, 18, 142

headaches, 4, 25, 83, 154, 165–166

heart disease, 4, 46, 78

herbalism, 52

Hermetic Staff, 32

hierarchies, 5, 39

high performance lunch, 85

holiday, 122–123

holistic health, 43, 51–61, 114, 123

home, 1, 10, 18–19, 21, 26, 29, 32, 39, 41, 55, 85, 96–97, 99–108, 122, 158

homeopathy, 52

hormonal control, 76

hormonal equilibrium, 54, 56

human potential, 48

Humming Bee, the, 29–31, 37

hypertension, 73, 134

hypnogogic state, 46, 109

hypothalamus, 12

# ☾ REACH FOR THE MOON

*Llewellyn publishes hundreds of books on your favorite subjects! To get these exciting books, including the ones on the following pages, check your local bookstore or order them directly from Llewellyn.*

## ORDER BY PHONE
- Call toll-free within the U.S. and Canada, 1-800-THE MOON
- In Minnesota, call (612) 291-1970
- We accept VISA, MasterCard, and American Express

## ORDER BY MAIL
- Send the full price of your order (MN residents add 7% sales tax) in U.S. funds, plus postage & handling to:

    Llewellyn Worldwide
    P.O. Box 64383, Dept. K630-0
    St. Paul, MN 55164–0383, U.S.A.

## POSTAGE & HANDLING
(For the U.S., Canada, and Mexico)
- $4.00 for orders $15.00 and under
- $5.00 for orders over $15.00
- No charge for orders over $100.00

We ship UPS in the continental United States. We ship standard mail to P.O. boxes. Orders shipped to Alaska, Hawaii, The Virgin Islands, and Puerto Rico are sent first-class mail. Orders shipped to Canada and Mexico are sent surface mail.

**International orders:** Airmail—add freight equal to price of each book to the total price of order, plus $5.00 for each non-book item (audio tapes, etc.).

**Surface mail**—Add $1.00 per item.

*Allow 2 weeks for delivery on all orders.*
*Postage and handling rates subject to change.*

## DISCOUNTS
We offer a 20% discount to group leaders or agents. You must order a minimum of 5 copies of the same book to get our special quantity price.

## FREE CATALOG
Get a free copy of our color catalog, *New Worlds of Mind and Spirit*. Subscribe for just $10.00 in the United States and Canada ($30.00 overseas, airmail). Many bookstores carry *New Worlds*— ask for it!

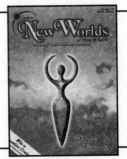

**Visit our web site at www.llewellyn.com for more information.**

Life is a Stretch

Easy Yoga, Anytime, Anywhere

**LIFE IS A STRETCH**
*Easy Yoga, Anytime, Anywhere*

Elise Browning Miller
& Carol Blackman

Easy Yoga, Anytime, Anywhere

Elise Browning Miller *and* Carol Blackman

Thinking about starting an exercise program but don't know where to start? Are you afraid that you may be too stiff, too old, or simply don't have enough time? Think again, because now you can take advantage of a basic human need—the desire to stretch—and use it to start feeling more youthful, flexible and strong within a matter of days.

*Life Is a Stretch* shows you how to breathe, stretch and relax through a series of simple routines based on the age-old principles of yoga. You can do many of the stretches in street clothes, at your desk, in a classroom, before bedtime—even in an airplane! Each chapter focuses on specific areas of the body such as the back, legs or abdomen, or on specific conditions such as fatigue, menstrual complaints and pregnancy. Improve your flexibility, balance, and endurance. Your body is eager to let go of the tension it has been holding for years.

**ISBN: 1-56718-067-1, 8½ x 11, 224 pp.**                    **$17.95**

**To order, call 1-800-THE-MOON**
Prices subject to change without notice

# THE OFFICE ORACLE
*Wisdom at Work*

Patricia Monaghan

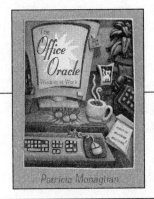

A strategy manual in the tradition of Machiavelli, Sun Tzu's *The Art of War,* and Tom Peters' *In Pursuit of Excellence, The Office Oracle* provides fast, savvy advice to help you skillfully master all of work's challenges.

With three quick tosses of four coins, you can become a workplace wizard. *The Office Oracle* will lead you to the appropriate lesson you need to ponder. Learn when you should smile and when to attack, when to take advantage of career opportunities, how to make money in the gray areas, and 197 other shrewd strategies for success.

Refuse to sleep through the marvelous flow and flux that surrounds you. Open your eyes to the multiple possibilities of every occasion. Learn to detect change as it is about to occur and use it to your advantage. Become one of the wise with the help of *The Office Oracle.*

**ISBN: 1-56718-464-2, 5¼ x 6, 224 pp.**          **$7.95**

## LIFE WITHOUT LIMITS
*10 Easy Steps to Success & Happiness*

Robert B. Stone, Ph.D.

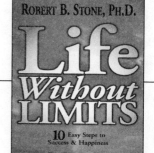

How is your life right now? Are there any areas where you still feel, well, quietly desperate? Help has arrived in the form of this playful and conversational self-help guide from Dr. Robert B. Stone. Dr. Stone is assisted by nine wise, but little-known, men and women who over the past 1,000 years left behind a valuable legacy for a joyful, desperation-free life.

The key to a life without limitations is provided in ten installments, each discussing simple changes you can make today in the way you do things. Sages from around the world will show you the timeless ways to make astonishing breakthroughs in all areas of your life. You will discover the culprit that acts to block your joy, and you will learn how to dramatically improve your luck...use body language to attract others...talk yourself into wealth...solve any problem no matter where you are...and eliminate the fears and phobias that hold you back.

1-56718-698-X, 5³/₁₆ x 8, 240 pp., softcover                    $7.95

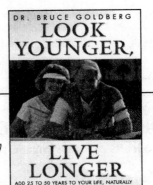

## LOOK YOUNGER, LIVE LONGER
*Add 25 to 50 Years to Your Life, Naturally*

Dr. Bruce Goldberg

Medical research has shown that your body's immune system is the most important factor in determining how quickly you will age. The key ingredient for keeping your immune system strong is a hormone produced by your own body called DHEA. Now there's hope for everyone who desires to turn back time naturally, without the use of drugs or surgery. Scientific studies prove that meditative techniques, including self-hypnosis, can actually increase your body's production of DHEA, knocking years off your appearance and biological clock.

In *Look Younger, Live Longer* you will discover:

- How to use self-hypnosis to increase your body's natural production of DHEA to slow down the aging process
- Easy techniques to boost your brain power and improve memory
- Nutritional keys to halt aging skin now
- Simple methods to significantly improve your sex life
- A step-by-step plan to reprogram the internal computer that may be aging you prematurely

Dr. Bruce Goldberg presents solid scientific and clinical evidence of how you can tap into the fountain of youth. Follow his recommendations and you will keep joy in your heart, a sparkle in your eyes and a spring in your step for many decades to come.

**1-56718-321-2, 6 x 9, 224 pp.**                    **$12.95**

## YOGA FOR EVERY ATHLETE
*Secrets of an Olympic Coach*

Aladar Kogler, Ph.D.

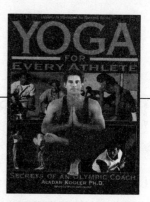

Whether you train for competition or participate in a sport for the pure pleasure of it, here is a holistic training approach that unifies body and mind through yoga for amazing results. The yoga exercises in this book not only provide a greater sense of well-being and deeper unity of body, mind and spirit, they also increase your body's ability to rejuvenate itself for overall fitness. Use the yoga asanas for warm-up, cool-down, regeneration, compensation of muscle dysbalances, prevention of injuries, stimulation of internal organs, or for increasing your capacity for hard training. You will experience the remarkable benefits of yoga that come from knowing yourself and knowing that you have the ability to control your autonomic, unconscious functions as you raise your mental and physical performance to new heights. Yoga is also the most effective means for accomplishing the daily practice of concentration. Yoga training plans are outlined for 27 different sports.

ISBN: 1-56718-387-5, 6 x 9, 320 pp., softcover                    $16.95

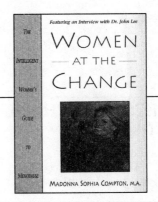

## WOMEN AT THE CHANGE
*The Intelligent Woman's Guide
to Menopause*

Madonna Sophia Compton, M.A.

What are the psychic and physical challenges awaiting you during your change of life? How can you use this time to deepen the quality of your life and emerge—like the ancient goddesses—a victor from the underworld?

*Women at the Change* is your step-by-step guide into the journey of menopause. Learn valuable information about the physical changes resulting from hormonal fluctuations, along with useful tools to ease your transition. Use the ancient myths to explore the often confounding psychological changes. Navigate your way through the controversy of hormone replacement therapies with the most up-to-date research done on synthetic and natural hormonal supplementation. Reference the most effective vitamins, herbs, anti-oxidants and phyto-chemicals, and read an exciting interview with Dr. John Lee, the doctor who is revolutionizing menopause by encouraging women to "divorce" their doctors and take responsibility for their own lives.

1-56718-171-6, 6 x 9, 288 pp., softcover                    $14.95

**To order, call 1-800-THE-MOON**
Prices subject to change without notice

## ECSTASY THROUGH TANTRA

Dr. Jonn Mumford

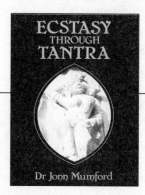

Dr. Jonn Mumford makes the occult dimension of the sexual dynamic accessible to everyone. One need not go up to the mountaintop to commune with Divinity: its temple is the body, its sacrament the communion between lovers. *Ecstasy Through Tantra* traces the ancient practices of sex magick through the Egyptian, Greek and Hebrew forms, where the sexual act is viewed as symbolic of the highest union, to the highest expression of Western sex magick.

Dr. Mumford guides the reader through mental and physical exercises aimed at developing psychosexual power; he details the various sexual practices and positions that facilitate "psychic short-circuiting" and the arousal of Kundalini, the Goddess of Life within the body. He shows the fundamental unity of Tantra with Western Wicca, and he plumbs the depths of Western sex magick, showing how its techniques culminate in spiritual illumination. Includes 14 full-color photographs.

0-87542-494-5, 6 x 9, 190 pp., 14 color plates, softcover     $16.00

## CREATIVE VISUALIZATION
*Proven Techniques to Shape Your Destiny*

Denning & Phillips

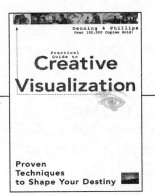

All things you will ever want must have their start in your mind. The average person uses very little of the full creative power that is his, potentially. It's like the power locked in the atom—it's all there, but you have to learn to release it and apply it constructively.

IF YOU CAN SEE IT...in your Mind's Eye...you will have it! It's true: you can have whatever you want, but there are "laws" to mental creation that must be followed. The power of the mind is not limited to, or limited by, the material world. *Creative Visualization* enables humans to reach beyond, into the invisible world of Astral and Spiritual Forces.

Some people apply this innate power without actually knowing what they are doing, and they achieve great success and happiness; most people, however, use this same power, again unknowingly, incorrectly, and experience bad luck, failure, or at best an unfulfilled life.

This book changes that. Through an easy series of step-by-step, progressive exercises, your mind is applied to bring desire into realization! Wealth, power, success, happiness, even psychic powers...even what we call magickal power and spiritual attainment...all can be yours. You can easily develop this completely natural power, and correctly apply it, for your immediate and practical benefit. Illustrated with unique, "puts-you-into-the-picture" visualization aids.

0-87542-183-0, 5¼ x 8, 294 pp., illus., softcover                    $9.95

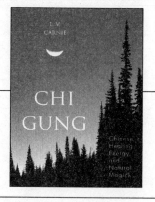

## CHI GUNG
*Chinese Healing Energy
and Natural Magick*

L.V. Carnie

*Chi Gung* is unlike any other magickal book that you've read. There are no spells, incantations or special outfits. Instead, you will learn more than 80 different exercises that will help you to tap into the magickal power of universal energy. This power, called *Chi* in Chinese, permeates everything in existence; you can direct the flow of Chi to help you achieve ultimate health as well as any of your dreams and desires.

*Chi Gung* uses breathing, postures, and increased sensory awareness exercises that follow a particular training program. Ultimately, you can manipulate Chi without focusing on your breathing or moving your muscles in specific patterns. In fact, eventually you can learn how to move and transmit Chi instantly, anywhere, anytime, using only your mind. By learning the art of Chi Gung, you can slow the aging process; alter your metabolism; talk to plants and animals; move objects with your mind; withstand cold, heat and pain; and even read someone's soul.

**1-56718-113-9, 7 x 10, 256 pp., illus., softcover**          **$17.95**

## 100 DAYS TO BETTER HEALTH, GOOD SEX & LONG LIFE

Eric Steven Yudelove

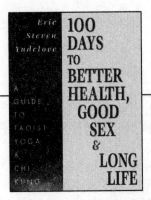

Humankind has always sought ways to achieve better health and increased longevity. To these ends, the Taoists of China achieved great success; living 100 years or more was quite common. Now, Eric Yudelove's latest book presents a complete course in Taoist health, sexual rejuvenation and longevity practices. These practices are not religious, but they are often quite different from what we are used to. And this is the first time that much of this knowledge is available to Western readers.

The curriculum is presented in 14 weekly lessons (100 days) that take 15 minutes a day. Each week you will learn exercises for the Three Treasures of Taoism: Chi, Jing and Shen—or breath, body and mind. *100 Days*...introduces you to the powerful Chi Kung, the Six Healing Sounds, Baduanjin, self-massage, sexual kung fu, the inner smile, opening the golden flower, and much more.

1-56718-833-8, 7 x 10, 320 pp., illus., softcover          $17.95

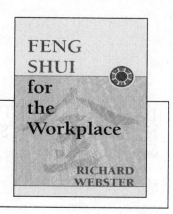

# FENG SHUI
# FOR THE WORKPLACE

Richard Webster

All over the East, business people regularly consult feng shui practitioners because they know it gives them an extra edge for success. Citibank, Chase Asia, the Morgan Bank, Rothschilds and even the *Wall Street Journal* are just a few examples of leading corporations who use feng shui.

Feng shui is the art of living in harmony with the earth. It's about increasing the flow of "ch'i" in your environment—the universal life force that is found in all living things. Chances are, if you're feeling stuck in your career, your ch'i is also stuck; getting it moving again will benefit you in all areas of your life. Whether you want to increase productivity in your factory, decrease employee turnover in your office, increase sales in your retail store, or bring more customers to your home consulting business, *Feng Shui for the Workplace* offers the tips and solutions for every business scenario. Individual employees can even use this book to decorate their work space for better job satisfaction.

1-56718-808-7, 192 pp., 5 3/16 x 8, illus., softcover          **$9.95**